BLACK PSYCHEDELIC REVOLUTION

BLACK
PSYCHEDELIC
REVOLUTION

From Trauma to Liberation

NICHOLAS POWERS, PhD

North Atlantic Books
Huichin, unceded Ohlone land
Berkeley, California

Published by   Cover photo © LanaStock via Getty Images
North Atlantic Books   Cover design and illustration by Mike Nicholls
Huichin, unceded Ohlone land   Book design by Happenstance Type-O-Rama
Berkeley, California

Printed in Canada

Black Psychedelic Revolution: From Trauma to Liberation is sponsored and published by North Atlantic Books, an educational nonprofit based in the unceded Ohlone land Huichin (Berkeley, CA) that collaborates with partners to develop cross-cultural perspectives; nurture holistic views of art, science, the humanities, and healing; and seed personal and global transformation by publishing work on the relationship of body, spirit, and nature.

DISCLAIMER: The following information is intended for general information purposes only. The publisher does not advocate illegal activities but does believe in the right of individuals to have free access to information and ideas. Any application of the material set forth in the following pages is at the reader's discretion and is their sole responsibility.

North Atlantic Books' publications are distributed to the US trade and internationally by Penguin Random House Publisher Services. For further information, visit our website at www.northatlanticbooks.com.

Library of Congress Cataloging-in-Publication Data

Names: Powers, Nicholas, author.
Title: Black psychedelic revolution : from trauma to liberation / Nicholas Powers, PhD.
Description: Berkeley, CA : North Atlantic Books, [2024] | Includes bibliographical references and index.
Identifiers: LCCN 2024012940 (print) | LCCN 2024012941 (ebook) | ISBN 9798889840626 (trade paperback) | ISBN 9798889840633 (ebook)
Subjects: LCSH: Hallucinogenic drugs--Psychological aspects. | African Americans--Substance use. | Afrofuturism. | African American philosophy.
Classification: LCC BF209.H34 P69 2024 (print) | LCC BF209.H34 (ebook) | DDC 154.4--dc23/eng/20240529
LC record available at https://lccn.loc.gov/2024012940
LC ebook record available at https://lccn.loc.gov/2024012941

1 2 3 4 5 6 7 8 9 FRIESENS 29 28 27 26 25

for me gente

ACKNOWLEDGMENTS

MOM, I HELD YOU AS you died. Now I hold your life story. You were the first to tell me about psychedelics. I laughed so hard as you imitated seeing trails at Hippie LSD parties. On those long walks home, you acted out all your Free Love, Young Lords, hot Broadway Girl hi-jinks. You gave birth to my art. Here, look at this book. It's your grandchild.

M. Noelle, you give me unconditional love. You give me *family*.

Son, you are the greatest psychedelic. When we hug, I rocket to the stars. I glue comets to my teeth like a diamond grill. I can love because of you. Chicken butt!

The People of Color Camp, you are my home away from home. You make a desert into a promise of a future America. And Burning Man, all of it, everyone involved, you are my Mecca.

Big up to Bed-Stuy, Brooklyn. You embraced mi familia when my abuelo, Emilio Castro Sr., took a banged-up merchant ship from Puerto Rico to land on your streets. Dear New York, you gave me love and pain, birth and death, loss and triumph. You get on my nerves, you stink, and you're expensive AF, but New York, I'm yours.

Kevin Balktick, thank you for your friendship and advice and love. Ken Jordan, hot daddy of *Lucid News*, thank you for giving me a map of our strange, beautiful world. Sia Henry, sis, you are so gracious and smart with edits. You saved this book. Quarry, bro, you treated this book like a man on ayahuasca. You listened and held space and told me what I was really saying.

Thank you, Jasmine Respess; you saw the creative direction I took and told me to go! You are the book's mom. And North Atlantic Books. Thank you for taking a chance.

CONTENTS

PART FOUR

Please note: The book in your hands is part nonfiction and part fiction. Some scenes are real. Some imagined. The reading experience is meant to be . . . *psychedelic.*

Such is Beauty. Its variety is infinite, its possibility is endless. In normal life all may have it and have it yet again. The world is full of it; and yet today the mass of human beings are choked away from it, and their lives distorted and made ugly. This is not only wrong, it is silly. Who shall right this well-nigh universal failing? Who shall let this world be beautiful?

W. E. B. DU BOIS

SETTING OUR INTENTIONS

BY MONNICA WILLIAMS, PhD

IT IS AN HONOR TO write this foreword for Nicholas Powers's insightful work, *Black Psychedelic Revolution: From Trauma to Liberation*. Dr. Powers is a deep thinker and a gifted writer. His literary talents shine throughout this book. He provides us with an exciting new vision of the unfolding promise of psychedelics.

I have been connected to the emerging field of psychedelic medicine and the mental health of people of color for many years. Currently, I am the Canada Research Chair for Mental Health Disparities at the University of Ottawa School of Psychology. My research on the mental health of communities of color involves work to ensure that everyone has access to mental health care, including innovations such as psychedelic-assisted therapies.

I first heard about Dr. Powers after he gave a riveting lecture at the annual Horizons New York psychedelics conference in 2017, called "Black Masks, Rainbow Bodies: Race and Psychedelics." Everyone was talking about it. Everyone asked if I had seen it. I tracked down a recording and watched it, mesmerized by Dr. Powers's insight and eloquence. We later had the opportunity to present at Yale University, and

I was loath to follow him on the agenda, feeling that I would certainly only bore the audience with my dry, scientific approach to the material after being thoroughly energized by Dr. Powers passion. We have since had the opportunity to work together in various capacities for psychedelic causes, and I consider him a great colleague and a friend.

Black Psychedelic Revolution is essential reading. As a Black woman, I experience life in a culture of lies. Our bodies are reviled and feared, sexualized, and exploited. Yet every corner store claims Black Lives Matter. Black people are strong, beautiful, intelligent survivors. Yet at the same time so many of us are ill from racism and the constant fight to prove our humanity to others and sometimes ourselves.

We carry the collective trauma of centuries of slavery, colonialism, segregation, and oppression. Here in the United States, violent methods of subordination have been inflicted upon Black people. Today, overt and covert acts of racism are daily occurrences, leading to racial trauma. The fear and hopelessness caused by racial trauma creates its own post-traumatic stress disorder.

Yet there is hope. Psychedelics have healed people globally for thousands of years. The West is finally catching up to the benefits. Research shows clear benefits when psychedelics are combined with therapy. Depression, trauma, and anxiety can be cured. In fact, over three hundred scientific articles on psychedelic-assisted psychotherapy in mental health care were published in the past year alone, making this a growing hot topic in the field. Psychedelics are different from traditional medications for mental health. They cause people to look within to find the source of psychic pain and provide insights for overcoming it.

Powers takes it one step further. In *Black Psychedelic Revolution* he carefully sifts the Black literary canon, sociology, and political science to show that psychedelics can spark a "Return to the Body." It is a traditional motif in Black culture and art. It drives a vision of mass psychedelic healing that can lead to rebirth and revolution.

Psychedelics are a tantalizing lifeline for Black people, but it is unclear if we are benefiting from any of it. Psychedelic research and communities remain mostly white, privileged spaces. Black people sit on the sidelines. If nothing is done, this gap will remain or even widen.

It is no secret that Black Americans tend to be wary of psychedelics, due in part to the stigma attached to illicit substances, as well as unethical psychedelic research performed on Black bodies from the '50s to the '70s. Back in the 1980s, the Black church was motivated to find solutions to the community ills caused by the crack epidemic, and in that process made an unholy alliance with the Reagan-era "War on Drugs." But the criminal justice system is heavily biased against Black people at every turn, from racial profiling to arrests to sentencing and onward. The War on Drugs became just another excuse to surveil Black communities and continue mass incarceration of Black people accused of drug-related crimes.

Because of the criminalization of psychedelics and the fallout from the War on Drugs, Black people face a great deal of danger when it comes to using psychedelics or even talking about them in a way that isn't true for white people. We have to be much more careful, and particularly those of us, for example, who are clinicians and are licensed.

Black Psychedelic Revolution offers a different path from the racist, sexist, colonialist past. Black people need the freedom and space to develop their own approaches to psychedelic healing, which may be a blend of Western medicine, community wisdom, and African and Indigenous traditions. The heart of this needs to be collective care and support for the healing of the intergenerational wounds caused by racism.

Dr. Powers is uniquely positioned to lead this conversation. As a scholar, writer, and activist, he spent years dissecting the intersections of race, trauma, and healing, making him deeply attuned to the needs and struggles of marginalized communities. His profound understanding of the historical and contemporary challenges faced by Black people, coupled with his ability to communicate complex ideas with clarity and passion, make him the ideal voice to guide us through this revolutionary exploration. At a time when the potential of psychedelics is being thrust into the spotlight, Dr. Powers perspective is not only timely but essential. He brings an unwavering commitment to ensuring that this burgeoning field does not leave Black voices behind but rather centers them in the ongoing dialogue of healing and liberation.

I am writing this foreword because the themes explored in *Black Psychedelic Revolution* resonate deeply with my own life's work and experiences. As a scholar dedicated to the mental health and well-being of communities of color, I have witnessed firsthand the profound impact of trauma on our people. I have also seen the transformative potential of psychedelics when used with cultural sensitivity and care. This book captures the urgency and promise of this moment, offering a path toward healing that acknowledges the many challenges faced by Black people. By adding my voice here, I hope to underscore the importance of integrating our cultural narratives into the broader conversation about psychedelics, ensuring that this revolution is truly liberating and inclusive.

In this book, readers can expect to embark on a journey that challenges them to rethink the relationship between race, trauma, and healing. Dr. Powers masterfully weaves together personal narratives, cultural critique, and his unique vision to offer a fresh perspective on the potential of psychedelics as tools for liberation within Black communities. Through this work, readers will gain a deeper understanding of the complexities of being Black in America, the possibilities for true collective healing, and the critical need to make these healing modalities accessible to all.

PREFACE

"WE TRIPPIN'." TIFFANY HADDISH STARED wide-eyed at her co-stars, Jada Pinkett Smith and Queen Latifah. "We trippin'."

The absinthe she slipped into their drinks had kicked in and they were *feeling it*. Jada grabbed Tiffany's breasts. Tiffany floated through the roof into the cosmos. Latifah hoisted hips on a Mediterranean Fabio who sported slick black hair. Well, she thought she was. Turns out, the Queen dry humped a lampshade.

"Yooooo." We rocked on the sofa, laughing. The giggles were belly deep. Our psychedelic lives were on Hollywood's silver screen. Our beloved Blacktresses took mind-altering chemicals, and it made us feel seen. The 2017 movie *Girls Trip* was a calling card. We replayed the film. Again, we laughed. Black psychedelia had arrived.

Everywhere I turn, Black celebrities are *tripping*. Mike Tyson told Joe Rogan he did DMT, known as N-dimethyltryptamine, and realized his greatest opponent was himself. Chris Rock breathlessly described an ayahuasca ceremony to Trevor Noah. He threw the gauntlet and said he was going to "break patterns." In an interview with Oprah, Will Smith described hiking muddy trails in Peru where he did fourteen ayahuasca journeys. In Denver at a major psychedelic conference, Jayden, his son, boasted that his mom introduced magic mushrooms to the family. Tonya Mosley from National Public Radio recounted a heartfelt journey through psychedelic therapy on her podcast *Truth Be Told*. Directors Ayize Jama-Everett and Kufikiri Imara made a Black psychedelic documentary *A Table of Our Own*. It is happening.

Black stars are talking publicly about pouring powerful chemicals on four-hundred-year-old mental chains and getting free. So one question becomes urgent. Can psychedelics free us from internalized racism, institutional racism, and intergenerational trauma? Absolutely. Can you hear heads explode in shock?

I know this is true. The effectiveness of psychedelic therapy has been documented for decades. First, in the United States, the research goes back to the 1950s. Second, psychedelics have been part of history from the drink kykeon in ancient Greek mystery cults, ibogaine in Africa, mushrooms in Meso-America, to LSD in the Hippie Underground of the '60s. Third, I know how powerful they are because of my own experiences.

Of course, there are risks. People with a medical history of schizophrenia or bipolar disorder can be triggered during a trip. Also, the reality is that unsupervised trips have inherent dangers. The drugs are illegal! So if you get busted, the effects are life-changing. Second, the psychedelic trip is a vulnerable state of mind, and shamans, therapists, and trusted trip sitters have been reported to take advantage. The threat of rape or sexual assault is real. Last, the chemicals induce a high level of susceptibility, which can lead to brainwashing. One can "trip" right into a cult or become a religious or political fundamentalist.

For me, psychedelics began in childhood. No, teachers did not dose my Turkey Hill milk before kindergarten. I heard about LSD on long walks with Mom. In the '80s, we were broke and walked to the mall and supermarket and back home. We walked so far that bus drivers honked at us on their return routes. Mom killed time by telling stories. She had been a '60s activist and hung with the Young Lords, Black Panthers, and the Hippies. And she did LSD.

Each step on the sidewalk seemed to take her back in time. Her face transformed into the '60s teen who protested, danced, and loved. I remember her playing the *Woodstock* album on the record player as she shimmied in the living room. I asked her about the festival. She had a warm, faraway look:

> I was dating a Black guy from the West Village; very hip, wore a cowboy hat, had his own jeep. He drove us to Woodstock and as you probably read, the roads were jammed, so we walked to the event, got separated in the crowd. For the next three days, strangers befriended me—me—this petite Puerto Rican woman. They fed me, let me sleep in tents and vans, gave me LSD and I danced in the mud, in the rain, made my way backstage, and smoked weed with musicians. It was the first time in my life I felt safe and loved, and it was by people I'd never met.

A light radiated from her face. There it was. The '60s. Whoever talked about it, glowed. Her face tightened. "We believed we could change the world." The spell snapped. "Anyway, at the end, I wandered around, and guess who I met—my boyfriend! Not angry at all. Hell, he had a great time. Even threw his cowboy hat from the car and yelled, he was so happy. And very chivalrous. He made sure I got home safe."

Psychedelics spark revolution. That was my first story. LSD was a sugar cube on Mom's tongue and the chemical key unlocked her inner glory. Joy and love melted the masks she wore to survive. Not just her either. Friends, lovers, and strangers took LSD with her and glowed like rainbows. The Heaven they longed for and protested for seemed in those brief moments, right at their fingertips.

I inherited the story of psychedelics as a revolution. When I grew up, I put that story next to new ones. In college, I read literature and saw art inspired by psychedelics. My favorite was "Howl" by Allen Ginsberg, which he composed while on peyote. *The Doors of Perception* by Aldous Huxley was turgid but sincere. I jammed to psychedelic-inspired music from the Doors and Fish and Herbie Hancock. College buddies palmed me tabs and we read the Gospels, watched *Jesus Christ Superstar,* and spoke in tongues as we ran the halls. Psychedelics were a cleansing agent, like a Brillo pad to scrub the TV commercials from my brain. I sensed deeper and more nuanced levels of life and channeled it into my writing.

What of psychedelic healing? I came late to that. After college, psychedelics faded in the rearview mirror. I was a professional journalist. I had a fiancée, student loans, and an apartment. The Modern Life Conveyor Belt had me going to Normal Town. In a rebellious spasm, I applied for PhD programs in literature. The Graduate Center in New York accepted me, and I moved back to my hometown in August 2001. A month later, jet planes rammed the Twin Towers. Fire and smoke billowed from torn steel. Office workers flung themselves from the windows. I stood on my roof in Astoria, seeing the dark smoke stain the sky, as inside, my uncle cried as the TV replayed the terrorist attack. The towers fell, and we all died a little with those inside. We cried and yelled and dragged ourselves through the streets, breathing ash and searching for loved ones with candles. We carried grief in our bodies.

A year later, I was invited to Burning Man, a festival in the Nevada desert, and when I arrived, I instantly wanted to leave. It was too happy. I was in mourning. It was New Age Hippie. I carried tragedy in my back pocket like a knife. Another New Yorker saw me moping, heard my New York accent, and knew my New York pain. He gave me LSD and MDMA, otherwise known as Ecstasy; he said it was not a miracle cure, but it could help. I gulped them down and took a long walk to the dark desert. The LSD and MDMA mixed in my brain. Stars fell like snow. I wept. I grabbed the dust and punched the desert floor. I forgave myself for not doing more. Rising from the ground, I walked back to Burning Man, clear, empty, and healed.

When I landed at JFK airport, I breathed and felt the ease in my body. LSD and MDMA healed me. They purged me of the weight of the dead. I could live again. I could imagine and love again.

Psychedelics can heal. I know that from history. I know that from my mother's life. I know that from my own body.

Can they heal us now? Yes, but how it can comes from a strange place. When the agent asked me to write this book, my first thought was it had to be in conversation with the Black Freedom Struggle. I went to my bookshelves and held *How to Change Your Mind* by Michael Pollan and *Black Reconstruction* by W. E. B. Du Bois, *For Colored Girls Who Have Considered Suicide When the Rainbow Is Enuf* by Ntozake Shange, and *The Language of Psycho-Analysis* by Jean Laplanche. They felt like pieces of a puzzle that had to be fit together.

What I found was a shared secret. In therapy, specifically psychodynamic therapy, one force really propels patient healing. It is Transference. The patient *transfers* unconscious wishes, desires, and memories onto the therapist. The goal is for them to realize what Transference revealed and reintegrate repressed material into their lives. I found this dynamic in the Black Literary Canon. It is in far-flung texts like Malcolm X's autobiography, the works of Zora Neale Hurston, and Assata Shakur's memoir, *Assata*. Except the crucial difference was that unlike personal therapy, the role of Transference in the Black Freedom Struggle was often Collective Transference that involved masses of people at historical turning points.

Once you see Collective Transference, you cannot stop seeing it. I pulled book after book from the shelves. Here it was in poetry, novels, and history. Even classic theories of Black identity formation, like Dr. William E. Cross's "Negro-to-Black-Conversion Experience," take on new import. Propelling the Black Freedom Struggle was Collective Transference, but it came and went, sometimes blazing in an all-consuming fire, sometimes sputtering like a candle.

Psychedelics in therapy speeds and deepens healing. Psychedelics in political struggle can be the chemical key to unlock the vast power in the masses of people. Repositioning LSD or MDMA, mushrooms, or ayahuasca as part of our culture of resistance, allows us to reignite Collective Transference. We do not need to wait for a Moral Shock like Emmett Till or George Floyd. New mass organizations could help us help ourselves by using these chemicals as a way of cleansing ourselves of internalized racism and complicity in the system.

For Black people doing psychedelics, true healing is not adapting ourselves to white supremacy, but we must undergo a new exodus. We must return to who we should have been. Our bodies are the promised land.

The books began to fit together. I saw the central thesis. In a way, I saw what my mother saw more than fifty years ago. She lived a revolution, in part, sparked by psychedelics. Watching her hands make rainbow trails, she was writing a new language that vanished before it could be translated into a blueprint. I looked at the piles of books, some new, some old and smiled. I had found a way to honor her life.

The joy of writing this book is that it became a psychedelic experience. Much as I plotted scenes and transitions, it took on a momentum of its own. Scholarship blended with fiction. Real life is warped by the gravity of the future. Dreams spill from between analysis. Holding it tight is a hope that we can become better human beings.

The book in your hands is a tab of LSD. It is trippy. It will get you high.

The book in your hands is also an act of love.

PART
ONE

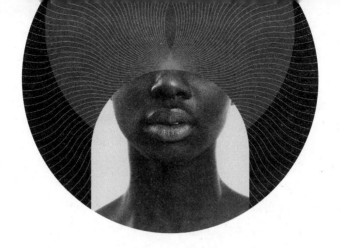

THE PSYCHEDELIC CLOSET

"WHAT ARE YOU WRITING ABOUT?" A smiling woman leaned on the table. "It looks serious." She pointed at my books.

"Writing about race and psychedelics."

"I *am* race and psychedelics." She jutted a thumb to her chest.

We laughed. I gestured to the chair. She sat and stared at the notepad with bright eagerness. Rainbow braids swayed in front of her small brown face. She brushed them aside and leaned over.

"I hope I'm not interrupting you."

Our smiles caught each other. I showed her *The New Jim Crow* by Michelle Alexander. Her almond-shaped eyes narrowed. After a minute, I handed her *How to Change Your Mind* by Michael Pollan. She held the books like puzzle pieces and sensed a big untold story would appear if they were fit together.

I asked her what role psychedelics played in her life. Steepling fingers, she unrolled her life story like a scroll across the table. Texas childhood. White suburban school. Teased for not being Black enough. Taking LSD at the prom and dancing, skirt above knees, one hand raised like an antenna to catch the future. Taking LSD with friends at a park, talking to flowers and hugging trees because "she felt the Earth spin."

"Feel the Earth spin." I laughed.

"Oh no." She gripped the table. "It's getting faster!"

"Hold on." I slapped the cup down. Customers shot glances.

She scooched her chair next to me, feather-touching my arm. More of her story gushed. Pressure had built over years to have a Black person listen, truly listen and make a part of her life real.

The elements of that young woman's story are the tip of an iceberg; it points to a shift in Black America on psychedelics. It is the inevitable result of racial integration, one chronicled in media personality Touré's 2011 book, *Who's Afraid of Post-Blackness*. The book is mostly a showy exercise in celebrity name-dropping, but he did chronicle himself doing white people shenanigans. One was skydiving. Elders warned him, "Black people don't do that stuff," but Touré wants "post-Blackness," in other words, to live free of the self-restrictive Blackness that is based on the fear of white violence.

So he skydives. He bungee jumps from a bridge. My man has no chill when it comes to being "post-Black." Yet Touré did not take psychedelics. No LSD. No MDMA. No mushrooms. Which is wild! Fun-time psychedelic use is one the *whitest* of white things to do. Of course, we know exceptions. I mean, who can look at Sun Ra or hear his music and think that man was sober? Yet overall, growing up I heard older People of Color talk about psychedelics as strange chemicals that caused whites to dance barefoot at Grateful Dead concerts, slide in mud, let hair tangle, and live out of flower-painted Volkswagens. When old heads said, "Black people don't do that stuff," my sense is they meant one could not risk vulnerability in a nation founded on and fueled by anti-Blackness. You can't let your guard down. What if some cop saw you out of your mind on LSD and shot so many holes in you that you looked like you wore a polka-dot shirt?

The young sistah at the café was living proof of the generational change between the Old School and the New School. It was the transformation that Touré wrote about, but she took it to the next level. She took LSD trips as casually as one would take a Greyhound bus. She was not post-Black, so much as post-fear. The respectability politics of the Civil Rights Movement, where activists marched in church clothes and painted the Stars and Stripes on faces to prove they were good citizens had transformed into *anti–respectability politics*. Instead of conforming to white, middle-class standards, a lot of us rebelled against it.

Why did this happen? The short answer is shocks to the system, massive bone-rattling historical events that pushed American youth further to the fringe. After 9/11 the blatant bullshit lies told by the Bush administration to wage the Iraq War exposed the rabid warmongering of the White House. Next up, the 2008 Great Recession forced millennials and Gen Z into barista jobs at cafés while paying off huge student loans. While making lattes, they saw that the American Dream was bankrupt. The youth fought back through a defiant fashion and lifestyle. They used elements of the '60s, '70s, '80s, and '90s white Counterculture from punk to raves. After being lied to so much by the government about corporations, over war, and about capitalism, they were just done.

The effect was that in the twenty-first century, a Hippie-sistah was as common as an emo-brother (Drake anyone?) or Jada Pinkett Smith singing heavy metal with her band Wicked Wisdom or a Black classical musician or a Black kid slamming in a Henry Rollins mosh pit or a Latino skateboarder or a Black chess player or a Black astronaut or an Indian comic or an Asian bodybuilder. When the young sistah at the café sat next to me, pulled her rainbow braids back, and tapped her multicolored nails on the table, I saw a casual experimentation with style, a gift the ancestors gave us.

We talked about the strange work racial integration had made of us. At thirty, she was a millennial, seventy years removed from 1954's *Brown v. Board of Education* ruling by the Supreme Court that made segregation in schools unconstitutional, sixty years from the 1964 Civil Rights Act that outlawed racial discrimination at jobs, and fifty-six years from the 1968 Fair Housing Act that prohibited racial bias in housing. She was the result of three generations of incremental, spotty, American integration. The Black Liberation Movement gave her freedom but also made her undecipherable to elders. She, Touré, and many Youth of Color not only lived cheek by jowl with white America but played with them and played like them.

And that meant psychedelics. Living in white America meant you saw its *wild side*. Underneath corporations, suburbs, and malls was an alcohol- and drug-driven Bacchanalia. It does not matter your zip code. It does not matter your class. In the tony suburbs, teens died of heroin. In run-down towns, Harley-Davidsons roared like chrome dragons in the parking lot as beer cans piled up at bonfires. You would be invited to orgies at a friend's house or to bare-fist boxing matches on a side street to a cheering mob. This is America.

Integration always came on two levels: formal and informal. The formal one was as you can imagine, the integration of work, church, schools, stores, and neighborhoods. If you are a racial minority surrounded by white people, oftentimes you have to be on 24/7 red alert. It means you wore your Sunday best all week long. You spoke your best English. You were watched. You were constantly measured and evaluated. You constantly climbed the ladder of success to prove you belonged. And to not let your family down. The stress of always being on display for white people and not accepted by your own people for being too white created a generation with impostor syndrome, always feeling fake, always like an Oreo, Black on the outside, white on the inside, or as one mainland Japanese friend called Asian Americans, "hollow bamboo." I was like, what the hell does that mean? She said, yellow on the outside but empty on the inside.

The flip side of formal integration was "informal integration." It is when masks come off. Maybe at a party, drinks led to sex, and the awkward moments afterward in the school hallway. Maybe after work, talk with a coworker at the bar spilled into rage at the boss or despair as a parent slid into dementia. Between classes, a friend said they had a friend who had Molly. You were invited to off-road areas to smoke and drink as car headlights stretched like gangplanks from a pirate ship and you could jump into the dark. You even found yourself at a heavy metal concert. What mattered is you were invited to places without rules. The test of being "American" was how you handled freedom.

Psychedelics are a glowing door in this "other" America. The more that Black, Latino, Asian, and Native people integrated white neighborhoods, specifically liberal ones, the more we were invited to Counter-Cultural spaces. Every once in a while, we were handed a tiny tab of LSD. It shone like a magic portal, and one by one, we passed through it. The sistah at the café told me her story. Now celebrities we grew up with and look up to are telling theirs too. The theme that unites their testimonials is healing.

Today, more and more are stepping out of the psychedelic closet. They bring stories of weird and wild visions, sometimes spiritual revelations, sometimes self-forgiveness, and healing. The question is quickly becoming, What kind of healing and for whom? How does it connect to the centuries-long Black Freedom Struggle?

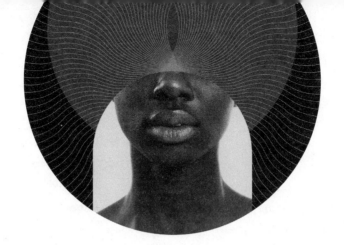

TEARS OF A CLOWN

"I'M DOING AYAHUASCA," CHRIS ROCK told Trevor Noah on *The Daily Social Distancing Show*, "with a shaman and the whole thing. I'm going deep, Trevor. Deep!"

He prefaced the admission by outlining his seven-hours-a-week mental health routine. Rock employs two therapists, a learning specialist, and goes to group counseling. Psychedelics, in this case ayahuasca, is one part of a total healing package to end toxic life "patterns."

Rock described the behaviors in a *CBS Sunday Morning* interview with Gayle King. "I wasn't kind, sometimes I wasn't listening, and sometimes I was selfish." He told Howard Stern that he was brutally bullied by white students and staff at the school in Bed-Stuy. In a sad and jokey voice, he said, "I was a nigger, and I got my ass beat. I got physically fucked up. Sometimes some sexual shit happened. I wasn't raped but rape-ish."

Hearing that makes sense. Rock forged mental armor to protect himself. The hard-edged persona of a street-smart comedian was a military tank he used to roll over the childhood trauma. Decades later, after he became the GOAT of comedy and after his divorce, Rock asked if that persona was now a prison.

Here is the paradox. Racial and class trauma follow upwardly mobile People of Color from barrios and ghettos to the suburbs. In liberal white spaces, informal integration leads to the sharing of drugs, music, and the white Counterculture. Yet those "liberal white spaces" are made possible by the historic oppression of People of Color, in particular the working class and poor. A few of us ride the coattails of white privilege and experiment with psychedelics. In Rock's case, it was ayahuasca. Others find LSD or magic mushrooms a.k.a. psilocybin. Whatever the specific drug, the healing happens far away from the masses of people who need it most.

In a November 2020 episode of *Red Table Talk*, a series of conversations hosted by Jada Pinkett Smith and guest hosted by her famous husband, Will Smith, he made a confession. At the Red Table with Dr. Ramani Durvasula, Smith said, "My father was violent in my house. So a part of the whole creation of Will Smith—the joking, fun, silly—was to make sure my father was entertained enough not to hurt my mother." On another show, he told political analyst Angela Rye about racist police. He looked distraught and said, "I've been called nigger by cops in Philly on more than ten occasions... White kids were happy when cops showed up, and my heart always started pounding."

The glimpse into his childhood culminated in an epic conversation in June 2020 with comedian Kevin Hart. Both men grew up in Philly, Smith with an abusive father. Hart's dad was an addict; he bandaged his father's failure with a strong defense mechanism, saying to Smith that it was "hard for others to bother me."

The two mega-star brothas nodded and parsed their inner worlds, hands moved in the air like men delicately defusing a bomb. Story by story they drove toward the truth. Hart admitted doubt at how priv-ileged his children were, and it made him worry that they were not "hard," or prepared for the reality of life.

"What my daughter is experiencing now is something that I never experienced coming up." He blinked and puckered. "I don't know what it's like to have a mom, dad in the house. I don't know what it's like to see a marriage on display in front of me. I didn't know what it was like for a family to sit at the table and eat dinner together or a family take trips. In my neighborhood where I'm from it's unheard of. Nobody had it. You might have been teased if your mom and dad was in the same house, if love was on display. What?"

The two brothas laughed in a rueful tone, sharing the loss that made them fight to be major stars.

"For my daughter." Hart made a prayer-like gesture. "You got this perception of how it's supposed to be, and it's not. But your conversa-tions can't be dream killing." He reached for Smith and then made a big circle with his hands. "Because I want you to want this. I want you to ultimately have it." His eyes scrunched as he pointed at the Red Table. "But this shit ain't real!"

Smith leaned in, arms spread like a gate opening.

"I heard a phrase called the Adversity Paradox. You grow up with a certain amount of adversity. You grow up with a certain amount of emotional bacteria." He bobbed his head like a boxer. "You learn how to survive with heavy challenges and heavy obstacles and bru-tality and lovelessness and chaos, and you learn how to thrive. You get strong. Then your children." His eyebrows raised and voice lifted. "And you say you don't want your children to go through that stuff. So you create a more sanitary environment for your children to grow up in. But when you take away the adversity, you take away the growth and the potential strength and development and the survival skills that come with that."

Hart made a head explosion gesture. Yes. Yes. Yes.

In their *Red Table* conversation, Smith and Hart exposed the conflict at the heart of Black upward mobility. Calabasas, the rich California town Smith and Hart live in, is a white liberal space. Top-level Black celebrities have homes there. It gives breathing space to heal childhood trauma from poverty, racism, and abuse. It is a new freedom, but it comes at the cost of separation from one's own people and ultimately the goals of the Black Freedom Struggle.

One example of someone embodying this intergenerational freedom is Smith's son Jayden. His music video for his song "Cabin Fever" showed him frolicking on Malibu beaches in retro '60s Hippie glasses with friends in tie-dyed shirts, while riding in a psychedelic car, singing about "tall palm trees and kaleidoscope dreams." Has Jayden done psychedelics? Yes! He said so, on stage at the 2023 Psychedelic Science Conference in Denver. He openly talked about his mother, Jada, taking magic mushrooms and introducing them to the family. Jayden said it helped him grow empathy and love for his siblings.

So, at the Red Table, the two dads, Smith and Hart, reflected on their lives. In therapy, they let go of pain or at least give it new meaning. Defense mechanisms learned in the street could be unlearned. For Smith and Rock, psychedelic therapy worked. It did for Lamar Odom, a former NBA star who took ketamine and ibogaine to end cocaine addiction. Latino hockey star Daniel Carcillo used ayahuasca treatments to rewire a brain knocked into jelly by seven concussions. Well-known boxing champ Mike Tyson took DMT and credits it for transforming physical and emotional scars into a road map of enlightenment.

Black, Latino, and Asian celebrities who integrated white upper-class liberal spaces are the first out of the psychedelic closet. They are not the first to do LSD, mushrooms, or MDMA. Nor are they the only ones doing it now. The difference is they have media platforms, status, and wealth. When Rock tells Trevor Noah or Smith tells *GQ* of their psychedelic therapy, they are borrowing a Medical Model narrative that began in the 1950s, when LSD and mushrooms were first introduced into Western medicine. Psychedelics alongside therapy can dramatically heal a spectrum of psychological trauma.

Again, the paradox. Is this powerful healing only the privilege of the elite? Is there any chance that the working class and poor can be given a chance? Will they always be left behind? What will happen if the masses dismantle the oppression that wounded them in the first place?

Kevin Hart faced that question toward the end of the *Red Table* episode. "We've come from here." He hunched over and made a square with his hands to represent the hood. "And we know how fucked up here was." He moved that square across the table to evoke his new rich zip code. "And now that we're over here, we don't wanna go back here and we wanna provide the best for our people *here*. But our people *here* have no idea, and because of that, when you do go out of here, which you will at some point, how can I prepare you as much as I can?"

In his phrasing lies the whole problem. He is there. He is in the rich zip code. He wants to prepare his children for the real world. It is time to turn the question around and ask, How can the real world be healed so we don't have to be afraid of who lives on the other side of the tracks?

How does it work? If Black celebrities are testifying to the power of psychedelic therapy, then what makes it new and different? Here we turn to an imaginary scene. Let's imagine Chris Rock on ayahuasca.

Hair in cornrows, lean and calm, Rock sits in a lotus position as a shaman blows sage on his head. Maybe it's an actual Indigenous man flown in from Brazil. Maybe it's a New Age white lady from LA. Either way, the shaman gives Rock a goblet of earthy, dank liquid. He stares at his reflection in the dark brew, stirs it so the image breaks into ripples. He takes a gulp.

In Rock's stomach, ayahuasca is absorbed; the chemical speeds through arteries, veins, and capillaries. Pumped to the head, the tiny molecules breach the blood-brain barrier and soak neurons, tangled like a ball of blinking Christmas lights. Inside his brain, childhood abuse is locked in loops. He built a personality around it like an Abrams tank, but decades later he realizes he is the one trapped. The ayahuasca ignites neurons that glow white hot and melt that persona like dripping steel. The trauma bubbles raw and hot. It will be experienced again in all its fresh pain but also "re-coded," integrated into a new, larger story that puts him in control of his life.

Rock comes at it like a pro. Whether or not he knows the terms *Set* and *Setting*, he and the shaman prep the scene. In psychedelic parlance, the Set is the mindset preceding the drug—maybe it's a rite of passage or artistic inspiration or therapy. The Setting is the physical locale, maybe a forest or a doctor's office or a mellow vibe pad with Herbie Hancock's *Thrust* playing or Alexa playing soothing ocean waves or rain on the windowsill.

Combined, Set and Setting can powerfully focus the trip. Yet a third term must be emphasized, *Container*. Ideology or one's cultural beliefs that preexist the trip also interpret its meaning. The wrong Container can throw the healing off course. Imagine a religious devotee believing after a psychedelic trip that God talks to them directly. What if they think they are God? The Container is just as important as the Set or Setting; otherwise one risks megalomania as in imagining they are Jesus, Quetzalcoatl, or the Big Bang.

When Rock told Noah on *The Daily Social Distancing Show* that he was "going deep" to break patterns, he already had the Container of therapy. Which meant the rising emotions would be poured into the sequence of Transference and integration that is established in psychodynamic deep psychology. The difference is he would go through it more intensely and at greater speed. Imagine those scenes in *Star Trek* where the ships blast into warp drive and stars stretch into pencil thin lines of light. That kind of intense.

But what does Chris Rock on ayahuasca look like? Well, imagine him drinking the goblet of grainy liquid. He lays on the mat. The shaman beats a drum like a heartbeat. Nausea hits. The stomach clenches. He was told the plant will forcefully clean him of toxicity and that he should surrender to the purge. Sweat beads his forehead. Trembling, crawling on weak arms he pukes in the bucket.

"Listen to the plant." The shaman beats the drum.

"It's very loud!" Rock rolls on his back and feels an electric hum zap each atom. His conscious self goes poof! Walls stretch like rubber bands. The sun turns like a crystal wheel. Breath washes through him and inner tides toss the mind. "Chris Rock" is now a spirit untethered and hovering in the wind.

"Go in." The shaman beats a slower rhythm.

Rock fumbles for his lips. "I can take my mouth off." He throws it like a frisbee. The mouth is a fluorescent ball that bounces wall to wall. It breaks like an egg into pieces, and out pops the white kids who tortured Rock as a boy in Bed-Stuy.

"No, no, no." The white boys whip out dicks and pee. The urine melts Rock. Inside him grows a monstrous-sized shadow that picks up a microphone. It spits fire on the white boys, who scream and melt. Shadow Rock watches as Madison Square Garden grows around it and encircles it, but the windows have prison bars. It can't get out. In the seats are white faces from his childhood. Shadow Rock laughs fire, and they sizzle. Flames char the walls and weaken the roof. Madison Square Garden is going to fall. In the audience, his parents yell his name. Shadow Rock sees them waving, and the flames dry into giant rose petals that float down. His mom and dad are two roses as tall as streetlights. They bend to Shadow Rock and kiss him. They apologize for busing him to the white school and peel off his shadow skin. Underneath is eleven-year-old Rock, scared and crying. The parent-flowers hug him. First his finger, then hand, then chest and torso and legs crumble into pollen, blowing away. He flies up, up, up.

Six hours have passed since Rock drank ayahuasca. The humming recedes. Thoughts crystallize.

Rock palms his chest. Blinded by tears, he reaches out, hands circling air. The shaman hugs him, and years of pain burst free. Gasping for air, Rock leans back and releases a roar of joy, and exhaustion, and freedom.

Now is this what happened? Who knows. It is a fiction, culled from Rock's ayahuasca trips and his biography. What is real is that we know psychedelics hurled a wounded mind through its inner Hell to emerge a more complete, more integrated, and more cleansed soul. One of the most powerful comedians in history is telling us that psychedelic therapy works.

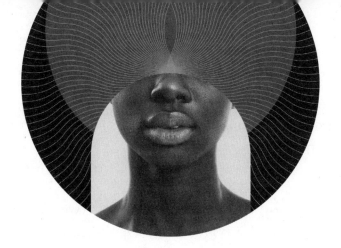

LSD AND AFRICA

"I TOOK SOME ACID ONCE," Richard Pryor told fans at West Hollywood's Roxy Theater. "White dude gave me some. At a party. He said, 'This is far-out.'" Knowing giggles rose. "I said, 'Well give me the shit, motherfucker.'" Pryor mimed chewing LSD. "That ain't shit." Affecting the white man's nasal tone: "It'll have you trippin'!" Laughter spiked into cackling.

Forty-three years before Chris Rock told Trevor Noah he planned a date with ayahuasca to go "deep," the greatest comedian of all time strode on stage and regaled ticket buyers with a story about his far-out LSD trip. "Acid" is the eighth track on Pryor's 1976 album *Bicentennial Nigger* which won a Grammy in 1977 for Best Comedy Album, in part because this skit captured the spirit of post '68 America. Drug burnt. Hedonistic. Feeling itself. Funny as it was, the skit did not capture the truth about Pryor, a man seen as "the voice of Black America."

Pryor's LSD trip is a perfect example of the importance of Set, Setting, and Container. As a gentle reminder, Set is the physical place, Setting is the mindset of the trip, and Container is the ideology through which the trip is interpreted. To say the least, no real therapeutic sequence was present. The absence left one of the earliest and most public documents about Black psychedelic use, hilarious but oddly vacant. The transformative power was untapped, which was particularly tragic in Pryor's case because the man was driven to greatness by pain but also destroyed by it.

Pryor was born in 1940 at his grandmother's brothel. Drunk mom worked johns. The dad, a former boxer, pimped and hustled. Mom vanished. Pryor's grandma beat him like a punching bag. He was molested at seven. Before reaching his teenage years, deep parts of him were shattered glass. Pryor could briefly leave that hurt behind as he walked on stage. He used the "Pryor" that the audience saw to bandage a broken childhood.

With that backstory, you would think the "Acid" skit would be a powerful psychological breakthrough, a journey into the mirror to heal. It just isn't. Contrast it against the skit "Africa" on his 1982 album *Live on the Sunset Strip*, in which no psychedelics are present but Pryor metamorphoses before thousands of people into a man who fell in wide-eyed love with Kenya and embraced Blackness. The two skits show that LSD has the potential to salve trauma but only if connected to a practice.

Let's turn to the skit.

"Twenty minutes later I was at the party," Pryor said. "Hey, blood, what's happening? Aww, man, ain't nothin' to it. White dude gave me some shit, talkin' 'bout I'm gonna be tripping. I ain't going no place without my luggage." The audience roared as he grasped at glowing trails. "Hey, man, look at this! I can catch my hands!" Pryor mimicked a high-pitched alarm as if the acid cranked his brain to level ten. "Oh shit." He spoke in a robotic slow-motion drawl. "I got to get the fuck out of here."

Someone in the audience howled in giddy recognition. "I can't breathe. I don't remember how to breathe." More clapping. In the nasal white-man tone, Pryor said, "I told you it was far-out!" A brief lull and then he despaired, "I'mon die. I'mon die. I'mon die." Pryor launched into a cliché, half gibberish Native American chant repeating, "I'mon die." Shoulders and hips undulated as he danced like an Indigenous warrior. "What in the fuck is happening to me?"

Pryor then held up his arms as if floating in space. He said, "Open the pod doors, HAL." The pompous trumpet horns from *2001: A Space Odyssey* blared. The crowd hushed in disbelief at where the skit had gone. Stanley Kubrick's film was a big deal in 1968. Millions saw the fight between astronaut Dave and the artificially intelligent computer HAL 9000. Now Pryor panted like Dave deactivating HAL and then switched to voicing HAL. "Please, Dave, don't, Dave. I'm losing my mind." More panting. "Hi, my name is HAL 9000 . . . My teacher taught me a song. Would you like to hear it, Dave? Daisy. Daaaaisy. Givvve meee yourrr answerrrr doooo . . ." A pause, Pryor ended, "Took me five years to come down off of that shit." Wild cheers. The comedian brought home an LSD experience many had but few talked about. He let them embrace, through his art, a part of their own lives.

Pryor probably did not do an Indigenous chant or hallucinate he was an astronaut during his actual LSD trip. The point was, his modern persona had been peeled like an orange and raw truth oozed free. Yet he did not perform his own past. When he chanted like an Indian, it was a symbolic unmasking of the fake self, and underneath was a cliché image of a precolonial Native. It made visible our internalized racism and complicity with white supremacy. When he played the astronaut Dave unplugging HAL, it was a classic allegory of the struggle between humanity and our programming by capitalism. When HAL died, and Pryor came back to his own voice, one can read it as a man reclaiming himself from the social machine to be his authentic self again.

As brilliant as "Acid" is as stand-up, it does not show any real transformation of Pryor. It is striking to contrast it with his "Africa" skit, five years later. In it, Pryor recounts his Kenyan vacation. It was a once-in-a-lifetime change. No psychedelics. No official therapy. Yet without either of those tools, he made clear that Black American consciousness needs to address cultural trauma to heal and fight white supremacy.

In the 1982 stand-up special *Live on the Sunset Strip*, Pryor paced the stage. Lit by a bright spotlight that made his black shirt and shiny red suit look like a Pan-African flag. One hand on the mic, the other flew like he was an orchestra conductor playing subconscious notes. He faced the audience.

"I went to Africa. I went to the Motherland to find my roots! Seven-hundred-million Black people. Not one of them motherfuckers knew me," he opened. "I went to the Motherland. It was so beautiful, just seeing Black people in charge of everything. I'm talking about from the wino to the president. It was Black. Blue-Black." The first muttering laugh rippled through the audience. "Original Black." Louder guffaws. "The kind of Black where you go . . . Black!" Pryor gestured as if seeing the world for the first time. "And it's great to walk down the street in Africa because a Black person in Africa reminds me of somebody here. I was like, 'that motherfucker look like Joe Frazier!' . . . And he be the president of the bank!" He stood in the spotlight as if receiving a message from the ancestors. "And winos that I knew here. I see them there and they'd be diplomats and shit! I'd be like Willy the Wino! Look at this motherfucker! That's what he's supposed to be! And you see the women are the most beautiful, elegant people, like *Vogue* magazine and shit be trying to work on that shit for years just to stand like these people, right? You be looking, and my eyes was full, Jack. I was like goddamn." Whistling and cheers swept the stage, and the tone was gratitude that Pryor saw Black beauty, and you sensed the crowd hoped the new-found love for Africa could begin to heal his troubled life.

"Cause in my mind, I figured Africa is a lot of jungle and shit, you know . . . Tarzan," Muted giggles. "Tarzan wouldn't last a week in Africa."

Big laughs erupted. "Oh, they probably just call him old crazy white man." Pryor imitated a Kenyan accent. "Oh, you mean the crazy white man. He's back up in the trees with the baboons." He asked in his regular American voice. "Is Jane with him?" And switched back to the Kenyan voice. "No, she's hoeing in Nairobi." The audience roared loudly, clapping and cheering.

Pryor's transformation in "Africa" showed that American racism poisons the mind, but Black love cures it. The skit began with realizing the beauty of Africa and the power it had to regenerate his imagination. It uncannily follows the work done by Dr. William E. Cross in his 1971 essay in *Black World* magazine, "The Negro-to-Black Conversion Experience: Toward a Black Liberation," where he sequenced the stages of Black identity formation. It was published eleven years before Pryor's bit on Africa and predicted his change. It looks quaint: on the page you see a Black man in a '70s corporate suit magically transformed, as if he rubbed a genie's lamp and was granted the wish of becoming a big-afro-sporting Soul Brother, ready to fight for the people.

The "Negro-to-Black Conversion Experience" has five stages, which begin with helpless internalized racism and end with a militant defense of all oppressed people. The first stage is Pre-Encounter, or when your mind is a warped mirror, reflecting white supremacy, you attack your own body. You attack Black folks. Second is Encounter, or some Moral Shock that shatters the warped mirror. In the third stage, Immersion, one dons Blackness like shining armor and wages war against white supremacy. You march. You protest. You shout, "No justice, no peace." Hatred of racism is worn like a Purple Heart. Next is Internalization, a kind of cooling-off phase where you strike a balance with new Black values. Fifth is Commitment, the final point in which a new Black self is driven by love for the long-term struggle and solidarity with oppressed people like immigrants, gays, and workers.

Pryor's "Africa" skit showed a man reborn as "Black." He went from spraying "nigger" like a machine gun on stage to disavowing it. He went from joking about Black pain to dissecting whiteness. So what was he before this rebirth? How did he get stuck in the Pre-Encounter phase of internalized racism? One way to answer that question is to imagine a new schema going the opposite trajectory, say from freedom to slavery. Title it the "African-to-Slave Conversion Experience." Imagine if the Willie Lynch letter were real. (It's not folks.)

The basic dynamic of white supremacy is the systematic use of psychological alienation and trauma to sever consciousness from the body. In Frederick Douglass's 1845 autobiography, *Narrative of the Life of Frederick Douglass, an American Slave*, he says in a biting, angry tone, "I have no accurate knowledge of my age, never having seen any authentic record containing it. By far the larger part of the slaves know as little of their ages as horses know of theirs, and it is the wish of most masters within my knowledge to keep their slaves thus ignorant" (395). Later, he wrote of his aunt being whipped until skin hung like bloody rags. Further in, he recalled a slave named Denby, who had his brains blasted out of his skull by the overseer for disobeying an order. Here is alienation from one's body through ignorance and abuse and terror. Each new pain adds to the Grand Canyon within oneself, and there at the center is the master's all-seeing eye like Sauron's flaming eyeball in *Lord of the Rings*, watching you, watching yourself.

Fifty years later, the founder of Black studies, W. E. B. Du Bois, crystallized Douglass's experience in a formula. In his classic 1903 book *The Souls of Black Folk,* he defined it as a "double-consciousness, this sense of always looking at one's self through the eyes of others, of measuring one's soul by the tape of a world that looks on in amused contempt and pity" (694). Here is Black life under a scalding white light. Thought blisters like a third-degree burn. The mind is poisoned by anti-Black caricatures like the Brute, Jezebel, Coon, or Uncle Tom. Black life wilts like a rose in a drought.

Pryor's soul had been mauled and pulped by white supremacy. The man was born in 1940. In his childhood, racism was public and legal. He was twenty-three when Martin Luther King Jr. gave the "I Have a Dream" speech in the 1963 March on Washington. King's famous "Letter from Birmingham Jail" has a scene in it that very easily describes Pryor. He talked of his daughter, who wanted to go to Funtown amusement park, but it was closed to Black children. King said he saw "ominous clouds of inferiority begin to form in her little mental sky" (1895). The more you read about Pryor, the more you realize he was that child too. In Peoria, Illinois, he saw racism destroy families—lost fathers, overworked aunts, uncles that were winos and hustlers—who raised him at the brothel. Shame was followed, inevitably, by rage. He felt a curse was placed upon him and everyone he knew. It laid waste to men and women who should have been his shield and stepping-stone.

Which is why the 1982 "Africa" skit is such a turning point. You hear childlike wonder in his voice as he described Kenya. He had a front row seat on how Black life, so often broken in America, had been redeemed in Africa. Pryor glimpsed what should have been; it turned his anger inside out like a fist becoming a flower.

At the end of the "Africa" skit, he made a confession: "One thing that happened to me that was magic was I was leaving, I was sitting in the hotel lobby, and a voice said, 'what do you see? Look around.' And I looked around and saw people of all colors and shapes." Pryor spoke with hushed sincerity. "The voice said, 'Do you see any niggers?' And I said no. It said, 'You know why? 'Cause there aren't any.' 'Cause I had been there three weeks, and I hadn't said it." The audience was pin-drop silent. "It started making me cry . . . I've been saying that, and it's a devastating fucking word. That has nothing to do with us. We are from a place where they first started people. In Africa, right." Loud claps and cheers. "I mean Black people, we are the first motherfuckers on the planet."

No psychedelics. No therapy. Seeing Black people in power pulled to the surface, buried hope to feel at home in his body, in his people, in himself. Racism has tools to torture Black people, and language is one of the most powerful. In his 1995 autobiography, *Pryor Convictions*, he wrote, "I decided to make it my own. Nigger. I decided to take the sting out of it. Nigger. As if saying it over and over again would numb me and everybody else to its wretchedness. Nigger. Said it over and over like a preacher singing hallelujah." The slur he spoke with operatic finesse, one second a razor to cut an enemy or cut himself and the next a rabbit pulled from a magic hat. Now it was a link in a four-hundred-years-long chain.

For almost his whole career, Pryor threw racial slurs like dice against the wall to gamble for his freedom. When he flew across the Atlantic Ocean and planted feet on African soil, heard the flowing music of tribal languages, he found a Blackness that sparkled like a star-filled night, endless and wondrous. The distance between American ghettos and sun-bathed Kenya, where a newly independent people strode confidently in bright fabrics, was just too far and it snapped the chain links of nigger apart. The brother was free.

Such intense transformation has a lesson for today. When you put "LSD" and "Africa" side by side, you see that psychedelics are not enough. Therapy is also not enough. Since white supremacy cuts Black consciousness from the body, to heal, it must Return to the Body. It has become possible now for psychedelics to power that "trip" home.

Black America needs a new freedom because it is the part of the African diaspora that wrestles living as an embattled minority surrounded by a hostile white nation. The price of being repeatedly stolen, from slavery to mass incarceration—stolen from the land, stolen from loved ones, stolen from our bodies—is that we become aliens to ourselves. Black history taught us to survive by knowing when chains are being clamped on; even if they are sold by our own leaders, even if they are painted gold. Now we have to paint a new North Star in the sky. It just may have to look like a tab of LSD.

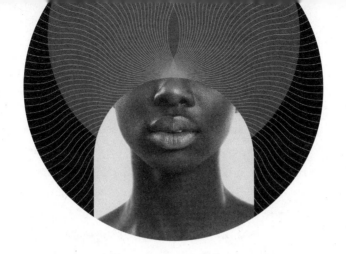

REDISCOVERING
BLACKNESS

"I WENT TO ZIMBABWE," PRYOR said. "I know how white people feel in America now: relaxed! 'Cause when I heard the police car, I knew they weren't coming after me." Laughter rose from the belly.

It is easy to say, "Well, the euphoria Pryor felt in Africa is lovely, yes, deeply moving but not relevant." "He said that in 1982. Get over it. Pan-African utopianism is done." Independence movements that freed the continent from Europe gave way to neocolonialism, civil wars, and genocides in Rwanda and Darfur. China ransacked whole swaths of Africa. Europe and the Gulf States bought fertile land to hedge against Global Warming even as the slums in Nairobi, Kenya, swell with the poor who tread dirt roads and live in rackety zinc-roof shacks.

What makes Pryor's rediscovery of Blackness relevant then and now is that *Blackness must always be rediscovered*. It must renew awareness of itself because the centrifugal force of global capitalism and white supremacy rips people from their land, their labor, and their bodies. The relentless spinning force that destroyed a whole people has been countered, repeatedly by a rediscovery of Blackness that like a seismograph spikes when the African diaspora erupts into independence movements and protests and art. Which is why William E. Cross's "Negro-to-Black Conversion Experience" is not a one-time event but *repeats in history*. Blackness must be rediscovered by the masses as a precious part of themselves worth fighting for.

Long before 1982, when Pryor fell in love with an independent Kenya, the African diaspora had fallen in love with itself. African people rose like a phoenix from the bomb craters of World War II. Protests against European colonization swelled from Algeria to Nigeria at the center to South Africa at the tip. Poet Aime Cesaire spoke beautifully on the human cost of colonization in his 1950 book, *A Discourse on Colonialism*:

> Colonization works to *decivilize* the colonizer, to *brutalize* him in the true sense of the word, to degrade him, to awaken him to buried instincts, to covetousness, violence, racial hatred, and moral relativism: and we must show that each time a head is cut off or eye put out in Vietnam and in France they accept the fact ... civilization acquires another dead weight, a universal regression takes place, a gangrene begins to set in, a center of infection begins to spread ... (35)

In a kind of psychological seesaw, the colonizer's sadism caused self-negation in the colonized who debased themselves. Cesaire wrote, "I am talking about the millions of men in whom fear has been cunningly instilled, who have been taught to have an inferiority complex, to tremble, kneel, despair and behave like flunkeys" (43). Again, the "African-to-Slave Conversion" in which the Pre-Encounter stage is in perpetual motion. It is a repeating trauma. Fear transforms thought to stone.

Blossoming like a rose from concrete, desire for recognition became a combustible rage. Africans demanded justice and police bludgeoned them. Shame pooled like an invisible sea of gasoline in their souls. One spark was needed. Whether it was a march scattered by tear gas and rubber bullets or home raids in segregated townships, all up and down Africa, explosions lit the night. Fires burned police stations, government offices and corporate headquarters. From the flames, new people emerged. Pan-African psychiatrist Frantz Fanon praised how violence transformed the psychology of the oppressed in his ground-breaking 1961 book, *The Wretched of the Earth*:

> The colonized subject thus discovers that his life, his breathing and his heartbeat are the same as the colonist's. He discovers that the skin of the colonist is not worth more than the "native's." In other words, his world receives a fundamental jolt. The colonized revolutionary assurance comes from this. If in fact, my life is worth as much as the colonist's, his look can no longer strike fear into me or nail me to the spot or his voice no longer petrify me. (10)

Here is the rediscovery of Blackness in revolution. Here are the Immersion, Internalization, and Commitment stages from Cross's "Negro-to-Black Conversion Experience" but with a turn to revolutionary violence to purge oneself of Double-Consciousness. After enduring theft, slavery, rape, and humiliation for centuries, anti-colonial movements from Africa to Asia to the Middle East were fueled by the knowledge that people are more powerful than death. The need to live and love lifted one beyond the body into a transcendent dimension. Here are the timeless principles: freedom, recognition, and love. Eyes met eyes through barbed wire and saw a truth, intimate and universal. We reflect each other even in the abyss.

Pryor felt the afterglow of this seismic revolution. He basked in it. The reverberations shook his internalized racism to pieces, and it fell like a dry husk. He stood on the land and heard the people and was healed. What happened to him would happen over and over and over. In fact, we just experienced it.

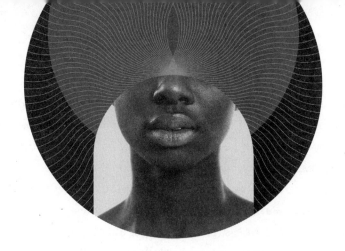

THE PRICE OF
THE TICKET

FORTY YEARS AFTER PRYOR'S "AFRICA" routine, Black America rediscovered Blackness in the face of a dead child. In 2012, neighborhood watchman George Zimmerman trailed a Black teen who carried Arizona Sweet Tea as he walked home from the store. Zimmerman bullied the youth, and they fought. A shot echoed in the night. Trayvon Martin lay dying on the grass.

When Zimmerman was acquitted in 2013, Black America erupted in mass street protests. The photo of Martin sprawled on the grass, a grimace frozen on his face, juxtaposed with him smiling in family photos hit that place inside where we love our kids and fear some racist could snatch them. It crystallized the cultural trauma, the story woven from scar tissue that ties us across centuries to ancestors screaming in slave ships or digging gold for conquistadors. The maddening terror rings in our mind. They steal our lives. They steal our love. They steal our children.

Against that Pan-African memory, Blackness became self-conscious. Martin's hoodie-nestled face was a bucket for pain that dripped from a thousand open wounds. Some so small or old as barely noticeable. Some so fresh and large they were endured by numbing. It could be the intergenerational trauma of drug addiction that destroyed family, or the self-surveillance at work or school, or shame at being too hood, or Double-Consciousness, personal racist attacks, or police bullying and police murder, trying to make a dollar out of fifteen cents, or cruel jokes by coworkers, being stereotyped as dumb, being tokenized as a victim, lied to, used and slighted.

Rediscovering Blackness in the early twenty-first century meant a new generation forced America to see trauma as political. The machinery of white supremacy—primarily the prison industrial complex but also housing and schools—set up pain, regular as clockwork, that either incrementally or in one swift stroke left trauma as a rite of passage. What is left is a vision of the United States as a nightmare realm, where, as Malcolm X put it, we are "lost in the wilderness of North America" and Bob Marley sang in "Exodus" for us to leave in a "movement of the people."

The Moral Shock of the innocent boy's murder forced many of us to see racism again as if for the first time. When you live in it day to day, it is easy to become numb. Skin hardens into an armor so thick that only severe pain can pierce it. Sharp intense pain like an electric jolt that zaps all of us through a shared nervous system.

As Black Lives Matter (BLM) crystallized, a double-front struggle was fought. The first against systemic racism and the other against internalized racism and the many morbid ways they reinforced each other. We began to look again at colorism, class, and crime under an unsparing light.

We joke about color a lot. We tease each other, play the dozens on skin tones, but BLM refocused our eyes to see the damage in the laughter. It goes way back. One of the earliest studies on colorism was done in 1939 by Black psychologist Kenneth Clark. He gave two dolls to a Black child, one white and one brown, to see which one the child preferred. Often they chose the white one. He and his wife repeated the experiment to measure how racism seeped into children and shaped who they valued or how they devalued themselves. In 2010, CNN repeated the Doll Test, with the same results. Colorism is one of the earliest signs of internalized racism, seen in the favoring of light skin and "good hair," whether from family jokes or dating or media bias. It leaves psychological complexes that sabotage one, silently, from within. So many tools of everyday Black life, from the hot iron to hair straightener and skin lightening cream, are evidence of this flight from the body.

Classism is the upward climb from poverty to working, middle, or upper class fueled by a contempt for those beneath you. I can hear the song "Movin' on Up" from *The Jeffersons*. Classism splits the Black Freedom Movements. Long-term solidarity is replaced by a reformist, middle-class agenda that ventriloquizes poor people's pain but not the revolutionary politics that would end suffering. In this fractured state, protests like BLM come and go in waves but don't build the power to topple the system.

Finally, Black-on-Black crime—yeah, I fucking said it—divides us. Bloods versus Crips, crew versus crew, Black or Latino men aiming guns at each other are, yes, driven by anger and pride but also trauma and internalized racism. They load pistols with the eighteen "fuck you, niggas" in the clip and one "bitch" in the chamber. They shoot at the dark figure seen in the mirror, and when he bleeds, they believe they killed what they hate about themselves. People are scared to go outside and ashamed of their fear. Parents worry about their kids being killed by a stray bullet. Kids idolize the power that gang members or drug dealers have. They leave home and come back with tattoos and ice-cold eyes. Brothers get swept into the jails. If they have kids, inevitably those kids are raised by the same streets that destroyed their fathers.

BLM not only forced us to see white supremacy with new eyes but also the damage it had done to us. A hunger began to rise to reimagine ourselves. In 2018, in a beautiful reenactment of Pryor's trip to Kenya, Black America took a virtual trip to the Motherland by getting tickets to the superhero movie *Black Panther*.

Sitting in a theater, I remember the movie light flickering on faces as we watched the Ryan Coogler film *Black Panther*. Many of us dressed up in Wakanda-Afrofuturist style to see it. A warm family vibe made us smile, slap hands, and make the arm-across-chest salute of the film's heroes. Rap stars even bought tickets for poor, inner-city kids to go. Millions of us sat there transfixed by this rediscovery of Blackness.

It was six years after Trayvon Martin's murder and BLM protests spread across the US. *Black Panther*, based on the eponymous Marvel Comics superhero whose real name is T'Challa, centered on the glittering, tech-advanced Central African nation of Wakanda. The movie smashed box office records, driven by a deep hunger to see Blackness as Pryor saw it on his trip to Kenya: as bright possibility.

During an interview on television talk show *The View*, Lupita Nyong'o, one of the actresses in the film, affirmed the power of projecting one's best self onto a lost paradise. Threading the needle between honesty about European colonialism and not offending white ticket buyers, she parsed words: "We come from a continent of great wealth but a continent that has been assaulted and abused." She arched her eyebrows. "What colonialism did was it rewrote our history and changed our narrative." Her hands cartwheeled. "Our global narrative is one of poverty and strife, and the wealth of the continent is very seldom seen on such a global scale." She made a large gift-giving gesture. "Wakanda is special because it was never colonized, so what we can see ... is a reimagining of what would have been possible had Africa been allowed to realize itself for itself." The studio audience clapped loudly. "And that's a beautiful thing."

It very much is. The beauty transformed moviegoers. The beauty transformed Pryor on his visit to Kenya. Black beauty. Black possibility. Black power.

While in the theater, right before the film began, I looked at brothers and sisters in *Black Panther* costumes and thought of my trip to the National Museum of African Art. It had been a year ago; I stood nose to the glass and studied centuries-old outfits and ceremonial masks from West Africa. Curious at a connection, I googled the 1895 poem by Black writer Paul Laurence Dunbar "We Wear the Mask." The first stanza reads:

We wear the mask that grins and lies,
It hides our cheeks and shades our eyes,—
This debt we pay to human guile;
With torn and bleeding hearts we smile,
And mouth with myriad subtleties.

The poem was a magnifying glass for how we hide our true selves to survive in the US. And that anxiety reappears in our art. Biting one's tongue at racism or clowning to ease white people's fears creates a rage that poisons us. Hiding oneself from the white gaze is a theme in the Black Literary Canon, and the mask is a traditional motif that shows up in poetry and novels, theater and manifestos.

The mask showed up again in *Black Panther*. Except here it sets us free. Masks give us a way to express our hidden selves. The film dramatizes this use of the mask in the opening scene when a meteor smashes into a valley in Africa. Pulsing with energy, it transforms the local flora. One man eats an affected plant and becomes an enhanced being called the Black Panther, who united warring tribes into the nation of Wakanda. He hides Wakanda under a high-tech hologram to protect the meteor's powerful metal, vibranium, from exploitation by the West. Again, the mask has a double meaning: a connection to a secret power and a way to disguise it from enemies. It repeats a traditional trope in Black art, where the central conflict is between one's true self and the need to conceal it from those that would destroy it.

This conflict tears families apart. Early on, a modern monarch, King T'Chaka (played with grace by John Kani) in the Black Panther suit, confronts his brother Prince N'Jobu (a pensive Sterling K. Brown) in Oakland. N'Jobu pleads that Wakanda must come out of isolation and rescue Black people oppressed in the West. He pleads with the king, "I observed as long as I could. Their leaders have been assassinated, communities flooded with drugs and weapons. They are overly policed and incarcerated. All over the planet our people suffer because they don't have the tools to fight back. With vibranium weapons they could overthrow every government and Wakanda could rule them all the right way!"

The king says no. They fight and N'Jobu is killed. The king hides the murder, but his brother's son, little Erik, watches them leave in a Wakandan jet. Let me tell you when that scene hit, the whole theater was so quiet you could hear a pin drop. Seeing brother betray brother to keep Black power a secret made us grieve and identify with the angry N'Jobu. And with his son, lil' Erik Killmonger, who watches the royal family leave on the Wakandan jet, abandoning him to the ghetto. We are Erik.

The other major theme in Black art and politics is that we are an exiled people in search of a home. We are lost and want to be found again. The theme can be seen in Jamaican Rasta praying to leave Babylon and go to Zion. Marcus Garvey bought ships for the Black Star Line to return us to Africa. Malcolm X demanded we leave "the wilderness of North America" and get our land. Later others turned away from the past and looked to the future for rescue. For example, musician Sun Ra, a pioneer of Afrofuturism, created a 1974 film titled *Space Is the Place*. Now we have Wakanda, a gleaming, sci-fi African city of tomorrow. All of it repeats a long-standing, deep mythos that, like Erik, we are strangers in a strange land. We want to take off the mask and come home.

School groups went to see the film. Families and church groups went. Kendrick Lamar bought tickets for poor youth. Millions of Black people filled theaters, popcorn in lap, and traveled to a fictional world that reflects our real desires. A new exodus was underway—not physical, but spiritual—to find a heroic Blackness, cleansed of racism that can protect itself.

At the end, T'Challa unveils Wakanda to the world and promises to aid refugees and the poor. He visits Oakland, where his cousin Erik was abandoned. He builds outreach centers to rescue the lost children of the diaspora. When *Black Panther* ended, a great cheer erupted. Our faces were bright. For a few precious moments, we were home.

Years later I can still hear that cheer and feel that warm family vibe. When we left the theater to enter the real world, our desire to return to ourselves and each other hit a very old obstacle. Classism and the gulfs it created seem unbridgeable. When we are honest, classism comes up again and again.

Let's return to where we started, Will Smith and Kevin Hart at a table, trying to make sense of their life journeys. They do not have easy answers. Just questions.

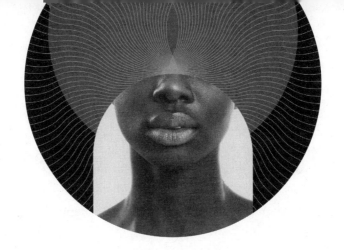

HEALING THE HOOD

"I LOOKED AT MY SONS," Will Smith said. "'Cause when they get to a certain age, they always want to test themselves." He shook his head. "So I made it clear, I was like, 'Guys, I promise you you've never been in a scenario where a dude really wants to kill you and you have to stay calm and you have to defend yourself.'" He play-winced as if punched. "You get hit in the face, and you gotta know you're okay. You've never been there. I'm going take it as my [parenting] failure, but stop squaring off, 'cause you don't have it." He smirked. "You were born and raised in Calabasas, and that's Spanish for *pumpkin*." Kevin Hart giggled hysterically. "So ya'll were born and raised in the mean streets of Pumpkin, so stop squaring off."

In the *Red Table* episode, Smith and Hart laughed at their privileged children, so privileged that the fear of violence was a joke. The Black Hollywood stars sat in Calabasas, which is 2,730 miles from their hometown of Philadelphia, a city that one month after their 2021 June interview was shaken by gun violence. Blood stained the streets like abstract paintings. Bullets cracked glass into spider-web fractures. While walking home, kids clutched hot pain, heard gunfire, and fingered torn flesh as a car filled with men sped off.

"It's ridiculous to me that a fourteen-year-old child can't sit on her porch at night," said Andrew Bey, a young Black man in Philadelphia. "I see my house taped off, I'm like, 'Yo, what happened?' They said a little girl got shot. But I got bullet holes in my window. Both sides of the windows. Bullet holes in my door." He swept up the shattered glass. "This is not the first time this happened. It happened like three months ago."

Bey's eyes scrunched as he stared into the camera. "I wish I was there. I would have taken the bullet for her." His voice squeaked in disbelief. "That's a fourteen-year-old girl!" He told the reporter that she babysat his little brother. Weariness weighed on him.

Days later, a thirty-year-old pregnant woman was shot three times and a forty-eight-year-old man was shot twice; both miraculously survived. By summer's end, 1,612 Philadelphians were shot, and the city was in panic. When the outcry reached a peak, Mayor Jim Kenney released a statement: "The local violence we are experiencing is tearing families and communities apart here at home, and inflicting trauma on Philadelphians of all ages."

There's the word—trauma—describing the pain throbbing after scars seal the wound. Time passes, but trauma stays in the body like a chunk of ice. It drips poisons into the victim. Anxiety. Flashbacks. Hair-trigger panic. Numbness.

Will the fourteen-year-old girl wake up at night sweating, her heart pounding? Can you see how that young girl could be silent in school? Checked out. Walking the hall, she floats like an empty dress, untouched, unmoved by life. You can see her grades plummet until she leaves school. Blown along alleys and streets, she drifts to promises of oblivion, huddling in playgrounds with runaways, passing a joint and cheap plastic vodka bottles. She lifts a hand. It is blurred, with a soft focus. Another swig. It dissolves. Then another swig. She dissolves.

Will the pregnant woman recovering from three bullet wounds become so numb that she stares at her newborn like the baby was made of stone? Will the man shot two times snap during dinner and yell or beat his kids? Will the EMT who hoisted the blood-soaked bodies into the ambulance see those dead young men haunting his sleep?

Here's the reality. Watching Black celebrities drinking ayahuasca or tonguing LSD is not enough. Living in Calabasas, the Upper West Side, or the Hamptons means wealth elevates one's "transformational journey" into a skillfully crafted spectacle, put on blast via media. It does not give a real chance to end racial oppression of working-class People of Color.

Also, if anyone in Rock's or Smith's old hood heard about their ayahuasca trips but saw Smith smack the shit out of Rock for a tepid joke about his wife's baldness at the 2022 Oscars, please forgive them for being ever so slightly suspicious about the supposed "healing" power of psychedelic therapy. If Smith snapped *at the Oscars,* what hope do the rest of us have? We have to imagine another world is possible, one larger than media celebrities. What if the Psychedelic Renaissance became the Psychedelic Revolution?

Imagine it's 2027. Reporters aim lenses and microphones at Chris Rock, Will Smith, and President Kamala Harris, who holds large scissors over a red ribbon wrapped on the doors of the People's Psychedelic Therapy Center. It looks like a five-story Christmas gift. Camera flashes create a strobe light effect.

"As I promised," Harris gestures to the staff. "The Mental Health Infrastructure Act of 2026 includes psychedelic therapy." She palms her heart. "After Covid, another Depression, another failed Republican coup, and reactionary Supreme Court rulings, Americans need help. Cutting-edge science can bring healing to minority neighborhoods. The People's Psychedelic Therapy Center is that help."

She cuts the ribbon. The staff in all white cheer and clap. Rock and Smith step to the microphone.

"We're so proud to stand here with President Harris." Smith puts an arm around Rock. "And to promote this center. Many of you saw Chris and I undergo our psychedelic healing in the televised special 'The Slap Heard 'Round the World.' If we can do it, you can do it!"

Rock leans in.

"Hell . . . I thought Will was on ayahuasca when he hit me." Chris laughs. "So when he said let's do a psychedelic trip, I was like nigg . . . " Harris shoots him a look. "I mean, brother." He makes a goofy oops gesture. "Haven't you done enough drugs? I mean I still can't hear out of my left ear." The staff hides giggles. "We discovered a larger purpose together. Who knows where a punch can land?"

Chris play-jabs Smith and accidentally hits his chin. Smith's head snaps. He blinks tears.

"You okay?" Rock theatrically squints.

Smith raises his palms up.

"Waited years for that," Rock says.

� ⋾ ⋾

One week after the opening, Nation of Islam, Five Percenters, and Black Israelites are shouting outside the People's Psychedelic Therapy Center. Glass doors reflect men in bow ties, rattling *The Final Call* or cosplaying people of Ancient Judea, thumping Bibles with fists.

"Stop poisoning the youth!"

"First crack! Now LSD!"

"Black people are not guinea pigs!"

A Lyft pulls up. A dreadlocked Black woman in casual business dress with a necklace of cowrie shells steps out. She steels herself to get through the gauntlet of hate.

"Traitor!" Spit flies. A Black Israelite lunges but is yanked back by another man. His bloodshot eyes and his knotted beard and liquor breath startle her.

"Judas!"

She walks like a bulldozer to the front door and turns. The protesters glare back. A question hangs in the air. Are they saving the youth from government brainwashing? Or is it a desperate attempt at relevance by Hoteps? In the silence, their eyes lock. *Look at you.* She thought. *You're trapped in the past.*

She goes inside.

"Dr. Iwosan ... " the staff cross their arms. Faces shift like mood rings, mixing paranoia, fear and silence. As the secretary leans on the table and the nurse fidgets, a thump makes them look to the glass doors. They see blurry eggs slide like jellyfish.

They gather. Iwosan leads a prayer and sharpens each word to cut home. "Remember, people who are most hurt sometimes fight healing. Hold on." She squeezes their hands. "Hold on."

She walks past rooms filled with therapists and clients: a therapist sprays lavender mist on a cornrowed Black man under a weighted blanket in one room; in another room, a therapist gives water bottles to four Mexican teens for a trip to the park; and in the last, an older brother cradles a weeping boy. She pauses at the door. *Good. Good. Release that shit.*

Iwosan sees her client sitting in the office. A puckered-lipped young sistah, baby-faced and tense, obsessively scrolling through her cell phone.

"Keisha."

No look. No response. Stone.

Iwosan leans back on her desk, pulls her dreadlocks back and sighs. Last night, she read the girl's file—thirteen years old, brother shot dead nine months ago, gang related—classic PTSD symptoms. Lil' Iron Chef here just razor-slashed a girl at school. It's either this or juvie.

"Keisha, do you want to be here?"

"Sure." A Megan Thee Stallion video reflects from the cell phone onto her pupils. "Free drugs."

Iwosan sidesteps Keisha and pulls the door open.

"Yo, you kickin' me out?" Keisha glances at the door. "The fuck!"

Iwosan lifts her shirt to reveal a dark scar, knotted flesh.

"I was shot when I was fourteen in Philadelphia. A lot of us were that summer." She squints as if reseeing the violence. "Hell, my neighbor made the news. I babysat his baby brother." She blinks and comes back. "Anyway, I survived the bullet but died in here." She taps her heart. "Did drugs. Did the streets. Did every mistake you are about to. Come back when you want help."

Keisha sucks her teeth and leaves.

❧ ❧ ❧

Imagine psychedelic healing centers opening in ghettos, barrios, and trailer parks across America. In LA's Skid Row and the hinterlands of Kentucky, white buildings with sunrise logos open doors wide. Staff pass out leaflets in recovery clinics and knock on paint-blistered doors to tell the poor and addicted that free treatment is here. People slowly trickle into the centers; staff lead them to large circular rooms where a doctor tells them, step by step, what a psychedelic trip is and how it works. For those who qualify, housing and food vouchers will be given alongside therapy.

After the trip, a patient may be found lying in a field of flowers, staring at clouds. Worried friends and family gently touch their shoulders. They wonder if their loved one is still themselves or if they got brainwashed. Chuckling, the patient says they learned how knots got tied and how they could be loosened. Turning to the bewildered, the patient asks for forgiveness or maybe they forgive their family for the stupid hurt they inflicted.

Many patients return home and drop love like stones in a pond. Talk flowed from kitchens, porches, and phone calls. Patients become like lightbulbs, their brightness lighting up rooms. When they laugh, it shakes off fear like laundry snapped in the sun. Some do not return, but move, choosing to find a new self in the horizon. Some question why so much hurt was visited on them, how did they get used to the poverty, stigma, and oppression.

A buzz is in the air. Something new is on the scene. *Hope.* Luminescent and fragile as a bubble. *Hope.*

Behind the buzz, doctors research their patients' records. They sit red-eyed at the desk, slurping cold coffee, reading charts, and prepping sessions. Curating music. Analyzing family dynamics. Cataloging key images and themes from prior sessions. Some reread Jacques Lacan, Patricia Clark, William E. Cross, or Melanie Klein.

On TV, reporters hold microphones in front of psychedelic patients like wands. The cameraman tightens the lens. Maybe the journalist hopes to catch a looney, weird spasm, or some cray-cray proof that psychedelics are a fool's errand at best, poison at worst. Surprise, always surprise, at a serene human being, deepened by an inner journey. Patting their chests, they say they feel like themselves; for the first time in their whole lives, they feel at home in their bodies. They stopped the meth, stopped the drinking, stopped the meanness. Smiling like a baby, many repeating the word "reborn."

Iwosan clicks open her browser and presses play. "He was a veteran . . ." In the interview, Rick Doblin talks to Joe Rogan. "He had been disabled with PTSD for years because of friends of his that had been killed, all the violence that he saw when he was in Iraq." He opens his hands like an origami bird. "Under the influence of MDMA, he had this realization that there was something good about PTSD. He was getting a benefit from it, which was it was the way that he showed loyalty to his friends who had died." Rogan hums yes. "That he was connected to their memory, and that he was suffering and it was a way to be bonded still with them. But then he was kind of able to see himself from the eyes of his friends who had died. And to realize that they wouldn't want him to squander his life." He raises a hand as if gesturing to the afterlife. "They didn't have life anymore. They would want him to live as fully as possible, and he realized there was another way to honor his friends, which is to live. And he thought, 'What am I going to do with the rest of my life?' And in that moment he cured himself of PTSD."

Iwosan pauses the video and remembers Kiesha, clutching her cell-phone, muscles taut as ropes, knotting herself around the memory of her brother. *She loves him. She loves him and can't let go.*

Rain streams down the window. Iwosan lifts her shirt to see the years-old bullet scar surrounded by the rain's silhouette. Against midnight skin, the shadow of droplets stream from the scar like the long tail of a comet flying near the sun.

I got you, Keisha.

⋡ ⋡ ⋡

Days later, a knock on the door. Iwosan rubs her temples at the desk, trying to massage the screaming from the morning's Hotep protest out of her mind. A nurse gently guides Keisha in.

"Glad you came back." Iwosan gestures to the La-Z-Boy chair.

Keisha is scared, skittish, and hopeful. Iwosan asks about her brother, taking exquisite care with each word like a burglar at a bank vault. As Keisha talks, she stops talking to Iwosan and begins talking to her brother. "Why didn't you stop fucking around with that crew? Why do you never listen? Why didn't you love us more than the street?"

Iwosan knows Transference had begun. Keisha aims her words in a wobbly way between Iwosan and then to her brother. It's like watching a player at Luna Park in Coney Island, holding a water gun, trying to hit the zombie face across the booth. She has something to say to her brother, and now is the time.

After a break, Keisha lies on the floor cushion.

"Ready?" Iwosan asks.

"Ready." Keisha nods.

Iwosan injects her with ketamine as the girl clutches her brother's balled-up T-shirt. The nurse spritzes lavender mist. The chemical relaxes her face, eases her jawline, and soothes her eyelids. Music fills her limbs. Like a sand sculpture swept by tides, Keisha dissolves. The inner talk shrinks to a tiny throb. She bobs like a buoy on immense waves.

Inside, grief is a jagged rock. She is dashed upon it and broken like a wood ship into a million splinters. Some huge hand lifts her, and there is Kay, her brother. He is a giant. She hugs, punches, and curses him in a spasm of emotions. He takes it all until finally he tells her, "Live, live, live. I want you to do what I can't. Live."

The ketamine hits its peak. She materializes. Bone and tissue, lungs and skin. Blinking back tears, Keisha looks up.

"I saw him . . . " An exhausted smile spread. "I saw him."

"He was looking for you." Iwosan strokes her sweaty forehead. "He wanted to see you."

⅔ ⅔ ⅔

"Your pain." Iwosan hands Keisha a book. "It's not just yours."

They hug. The young woman leaves through a side door to avoid the protest and gets on the subway train, glowing, tired but happy. *Turned inside out, I've been turned inside out.* As the train rocks, she closes her eyes and sees him there. He is a pearl clamped by a shell, plucked out and freed.

Home was strange. Now Keisha could see her neighbors with new eyes. She saw men and women hunched as if dragging chains. Prune-wrinkled men downed beers in paper bags to numb failed lives. Her friends bandaged hurt with the videos on their cellphones, dressing and talking like celebrities. Wherever she glanced, she saw bodies screwed tight to keep pain repressed. *How did we get like this?*

Lying on her bed, she thumbs through the book Dr. Iwosan gave her, *Black Psychedelic Revolution,* and the first line hit, "For Black people doing psychedelics, true healing is not adapting ourselves to white supremacy, but we must undergo a new exodus. We must return to who we should have been. Our bodies are the promised land."

Me? She palms her chest. *Me?*

≩ ≩ ≩

Not again. Iwosan rubs her temples in the Lyft. *Not again.*

The car pulls up to the People's Psychedelic Therapy Center. Face hard like a mask, she gets out and sees snarling Black Israelites and Hotep protesters. God, they curse her momma. Curse her to Hell and back. Before she takes a step, a phalanx of brothers, all in black T-shirts march up and stand nose-to-nose with the mob.

Iwosan freezes.

"You saved my son." The leader shows her a photo of a teen she treated for drug addiction months ago. "We got this."

Iwosan's feet feel stuck in mud. Slowly she walks to the doors as the Black men guard her. She knows them. Some are ex-felons trying to piece life back together, raise kids they hadn't seen for years, deal with PTSD, deal with shame. She met them at family counseling with clients. Sure a few called to say thank you, but she didn't think she'd see them again.

"Nigga, what you going to do?" A Hotep gets in the leader's face; he pushes back so hard the Hotep nearly does a somersault.

"That's what I'm about," he asserts. "That's what I'm about."

Fear drains the protesters' strength from them. They back away, cursing and scowling but leaving.

Iwosan closes the doors, waves the staff over to look, but they are transfixed by the TV bolted on the wall. On it, Florida Governor Ron DeSantis waves a copy of *Black Psychedelic Revolution,* "Now we see what these psychedelic treatment centers are really about. They're Leftist incubation centers, brainwashing Americans with critical race theory. This book was given to a client in one of these so-called 'healing centers.' It just teaches hate of America, hate of white people, hate of Jesus. Listen to this passage, 'For Black people doing psychedelics, true healing is not adapting ourselves to white supremacy . . . ' It goes on and on."

Phones ring at the desk. Cell phones buzz in their pockets. Staff palm their faces. Email notifications beep on the computers. Clients stumble from rooms into the hallway, take off sleeping masks, and stare, confused.

⋟ ⋟ ⋟

Imagine a backlash against psychedelic healing. Imagine Fox News reporters doggedly chasing staff with microphones, yelling questions as a shaky camera captures a panicked doctor dashing into a car. Republicans would call for the immediate shutdown of the treatment centers and a recriminalizing of the drugs.

As elections loom, psychedelic therapy could be the face of a new moral panic, a new boogey-man conjured by Conservatives. It would repeat the 1960s when LSD was first criminalized and portrayed as a gift from Satan, a seductive "trip" that ended in madness and left promising youth shaking invisible bugs from their hair. Except now, madness was caused not just by chemicals but chemicals mixed with Black history or Leftist ideology.

Patients who testify to the healing could be caught between the truth experienced first-hand and suspicious glares in the street. At a bar, a loud, boorish man, maybe a friend of a friend, would join a table full of people for drinks and accuse anyone who did the treatment of poisoning America. In countless conversations across towns and cities, lines to a concert, or at the voting booths, psychedelic healing would be politicized, ripped away from the reality to fit a cartoon image of mad Communist scientists pouring smoking test tubes of strange concoctions down people's throats.

Imagine psychedelic activists and doctors on Zoom meetings, despairing at decades of work to retell the story of psychedelics now ripped to shreds. Twiddling eyeglasses, one would say that maybe they should temporarily halt treatments. Why poke a bear? An awkward silence on the Zoom call, the air stinking of fear.

No.

A doctor from New York's Brooklyn treatment center in a business suit and cowrie shells, dreadlocks in a bun—Iwosan—is saying no. Too many retreats have been made already. Too many fallbacks. America is sick. Has been for a long time.

She tells them about a young girl whose brother was shot and has PTSD. After a ketamine trip and therapy, she went back to school. Are we going to take away her chance at a good life because rich racists lie about who we are?

⸙ ⸙ ⸙

Life.

Keisha leans into the sun. Her skin is like a sunflower, soaking light.

Life.

In her hand, sweat glitters like tiny seeds. Smiling wide, she turns from the window to the mirror. She pulls on her *Exodus* shirt with the Bob Marley Exodus album cover in bright yellow. Next, Pan-African wristbands, ointment on the new tattoo of a lion, and a pinky finger smoothing fresh cornrows. Total dap.

Black life. Seeing Black. Tasting Black. Loving Black. The psychedelic trip, the books, the Malcolm X YouTube clips, the political chat rooms. Yeah, some of it is cray-cray, some over her head, but it adds to the change, one a long time coming, a recentering of herself in what she actually wants—pride in her body and its history.

In the street, neighbors quietly put her on a scale. A few roll their eyes. Most smile and some raise a fist. Quotes from *Exodus* appear on

Black-owned barbershops. Once a week, speakers from Black Lives Matter stand on egg crates and say BLM is dead, reformism is dead, America is dead, the Earth is dead, and we have to leave, get outta here, Exodus time!

Keisha strides past the drunks; usually they look her up and down with their eyes, but now they raise bottles in salute.

"All right now." One wipes his mouth. "She a queen, now."

"We all royalty."

"Not all." He elbows a friend who has nodded off.

"Who taught you that?" She puts one foot on the step. "Who taught you to be less than what you are?" The words pierce the liquor haze. "Time to go, and we want everyone to come with us. That. Means. You." She points at each man. "I did that psychedelic treatment. At the center, lots of friends, addicted, got clean after a few sessions. Just check 'em out. If you are on Medicare, it's free."

"You grown." He puts the bottle down.

"*Growing*." She stands up and looks down the street. "Growing."

Outside the People's Psychedelic Therapy Center an ominous silence makes the heart tighten. Dr. Iwosan sees people on building stoops, huddling over cellphones, darkly murmuring. The combinations don't make sense. Church ladies sitting with drunks, MTA drivers with Hoteps, gay couples with hustlers; all Black, all sharing the same burden, the same shadow passing their faces.

She walks to one crew. A man hits his fist into his hand, repeating, "Motherfuckers." An off-duty security guard shushes him. On the screen, President Harris says, "Today's Supreme Court decision to overturn *Brown v. Board of Education* and the Voting Rights Act shocks the conscience of the nation."

Iwosan's heart kicks, and a dizzy spell makes her sit. *What? What. What. How? Why?*

⤳ ⤳ ⤳

The street is a held breath. Air is sucked backward and up. Nothing left to say. Nothing left to think.

Rage rises silently. Everyone feels it fall across the city. The hairs on arms stand. Scared people dash indoors.

Iwosan grips the windowsill, and from the street yells erupt. Glass shatters. The explosion begins. It begins inside her. Dizziness spins thoughts into a black hole that penetrates time itself. Memory kicks and punches inside her body. Countless enslaved ancestors crawl up her throat. *No. No. No. Life is not worth living in a living death.*

She runs down the stairs, the street, and into a moving river of people. Black families in doorways pour into the movement. Iwosan sees flames twisting from a police van, bright red, dry crackling in the eerie silence. In the dark, on every face, the fire is reflected in thousands of eyes so it looks like innumerable ignited torches fell on the city.

"Exodus now!" Around her, fists thrust into the air with *Exodus* tattooed on forearms. Iwosan sees Keisha and zigzags to her. The young woman sees her, smiles, holds out a finger with a tab of LSD on it.

"Your turn, doctor."

Iwosan tongues the tab.

"We're not going back." Keisha says. "Healing showed me the cause of our pain was thinking this could ever be home." She makes a sweeping gesture to America. "Its heart has hardened. It will not let us go. Tonight we are the pillar of fire. Tonight we kill the pharaoh." She hugs Iwosan and moves deep into the march, forever gone.

Iwosan feels the end coming. All the weight she bore upon her shoulders since childhood becomes measurable exactly as it slides off. Racism has been there her whole life. Molding her like an invisible sculptor. As a teen, she stood at the mirror and worried about her midnight complexion. Racism was in constant self-doubt. Racism was in her lovemaking when she ran through white frat guys in college to be rescued from Blackness. Racism was in her middle-class parody of "working-in-the-system."

Racism heaped the nightmare of centuries on her life. She thought it would just always be and hedged her bets to abide by it. Not anymore. Glancing face-to-face, she knows tonight, America is done. The people had been forced to see the darkness of slavery opening beneath their feet. Just one law cracked, and the Hell the ancestors survived reached for them anew.

Burn it. Burn it down.

The LSD kicks in and she climbs a streetlight. The people hit police barricades like a tsunami. Cops and riot shields fly into the air. Tear gas clouds twist around bodies like hands made of smoke. Thundering chants bowl up and down the avenues. Fire churns from the broken windows of city hall.

The LSD erases layer after layer of her ego. Holding on to the light, Iwosan reaches fingertips out to the brewing revolution and wipes her face, tearing off the mask that conceals her truth. Black love swells like a sunrise. And it feels good.

A loud explosion tears the roof off the police station. Fire flares from more buildings. This was it. They were leaving America. *Goodbye, baby. Goodbye.* The woman she had been to survive here blew away in the heat.

Feeling crazy joy, she cries and laughs. And jumps into the march.

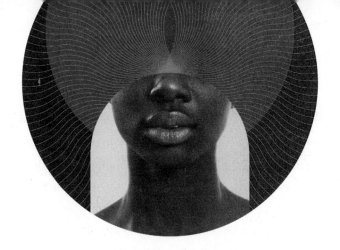

ANOTHER WORLD
IS POSSIBLE

PSYCHEDELICS REVEAL A TRUTH ABOUT ourselves. The healing that celebrities hail as life-changing and transformative points to a vast ocean of pain that exists in millions of people. They carry it from the past. They bear it in the present. They, too, want to believe that some relief, some rescue, can come for them.

It can. The price of the fully realized power of psychedelics is a revolution that shakes off the husk of the West and brings forth a new human world. It is not without risk. Psychedelics are very powerful and, yes, in some rare cases they can trigger a psychotic episode. The risk is mostly in those with a predisposition. Also there are real safety concerns. Physical safety is one of the risks. For women in particular, sexual safety has to be secured. Too many women have been raped or violated when they are on a vulnerable psychedelic trip. Last but definitely not least is psychological safety. The chemically opened mind is a powerful state that should not be abused by having it poured into the mold of a cult follower or religious zealot.

Considering these risks, the Trojan horse tactic of the current Medical Model does come with safety protocols and erases some of the Drug War–era stigma. It absolutely does, but the collateral damage is the revolutionary politics of the '60s. The many benefits of the Medical Model must be acknowledged but so, too, the fact that it chokes racial liberation.

For every Mike Tyson, Will Smith, or Chris Rock, there is a multitude of People of Color who suffer invisibly. They sleep in tents on Skid Row. They cook meals under highway overpasses. They work and work and work, come home wrecked and unable to feel love. They watch TV in jail cells, numbing themselves to the passage of time and the lost bond to children.

To be historically relevant to the twenty-first-century human crisis, the Psychedelic Renaissance must become a Psychedelic Revolution. Activists and scientists, identity-hustlers and New Age seekers must turn from internecine squabbles over money, as billion-dollar businesses monetize healing. Whole frames of reference, the rhetoric in play and organizational forms will have to be jettisoned to make space for a new relationship to psychedelics, and more importantly, to the raw, volatile hope they call to the surface.

In the 2022 Netflix documentary *How to Change Your Mind*, founder of the Multidisciplinary Association for Psychedelic Studies (MAPS), Rick Doblin, set the record straight on why he dedicated decades of his life to this single goal. He began MAPS in 1986 and it has become the juggernaut in the movement. I've met Doblin many times and admire him. The man has a winning, impish smile like a street magician. He is also terrifyingly smart. Just listening to him list off people, ideas, policies, and the countless moving pieces of the Psychedelic Renaissance is jolting.

Doblin led MAPS through the byzantine maze of the Food and Drug Administration to get MDMA federal approval for therapy. It hit a new wall in 2024 when the FDA did not approve MDMA and MAPS had to regroup and find a new way forward. What drove Doblin through decades of rollercoaster hope and setbacks was social justice. He said in the documentary, "My family is Jewish, and I was raised on stories of the Holocaust. I grew up with violent political assassinations. The Vietnam War was raging. The riots were happening in America. I thought if people could have this connection, this connection with nature, connection with everything, then it's going to be harder to demonize others." He looked into the camera, steady and forthright. "It's going to be harder to commit genocide. And harder to see others as your enemy that you have to kill."

Episode three of the documentary, which focused on MDMA, had a scene about Doblin's graduate thesis. Host Michael Pollan, noted writer famous for his best-selling 2018 book the documentary was based on, talked about Doblin's PhD thesis, saying, "His thesis, 'Regulation of the Medical Use of Psychedelics and Marijuana,' is the roadmap for the Psychedelic Renaissance. It worked. We are now on the precipice of FDA approval of MDMA for medical use. Following Doblin's playbook, LSD, psilocybin, or mescaline could foreseeably be legalized too."

To realize that vision, a new playbook has to be written that presumes legalized psychedelics and "maps" the next steps. The Psychedelic Renaissance is in the same position to political struggle as utopian socialism was to revolutionary socialism; it assumes public access to a quantifiable, proven good. In this case MDMA enhanced therapy can, on its own, attract the masses and elites into a peaceful, transcendence. Psychedelic utopianism is only now, after pressure from Black and Latino, Asian and Indigenous, queer and disabled, nonbinary and socialist explorers, edging to a fuller understanding of different healing methods that can reach more people. But it's not enough.

What is missing is engagement with the Black Freedom Movement. Also it must dialogue with literature and evolutionary psychology, socialism, and anthropology. The reason it must do so ASAP is because the psychedelic connection that Doblin hopes will end war, genocide, and prejudice must inevitably *run into a reactionary backlash*. The utopianism of the Counterculture is risky because it paints a false image of class conflict. Big Business will fight psychedelics if too many people envision life beyond capitalism. Politicians will recriminalize them if users see beyond propaganda and demand universal basic income, universal health care, peace instead of war, and the end of poverty. Yet the dream of a nonmaterialistic and nonviolent world is exactly what drives the Psychedelic Renaissance.

How do we heal the hood? Or the favela or barrio? Or the trailer park?

How do we heal Wall Street? Or the prison industrial complex? Or the Pentagon?

How do we heal a global capitalism that destroys the Earth?

How do we heal women who endure violence from men? How do we heal the men who are violent? How do we heal from binary sexuality? How do we heal from the nuclear family and monogamy?

How do we heal the very split between the body and the "self"? Is not the body the site of the original wound that we attempt to bandage by wrapping ephemeral imagery around the five senses? Are we not addicted to the ego? Do we not love the hall of mirrors that is other people?

ॐ ॐ ॐ

When the rainbow-braided Black girl in the café heard that I was writing about race and psychedelics, she hefted Michael Pollan's *How to Change Your Mind* and Michelle Alexander's *The New Jim Crow* and tried to fit them like puzzle pieces. She intuited that between these voices was a conversation she needed to hear. In the following chapters, Karl Marx visits the Oracle at Delphi, María Sabina hugs Michael Pollan, and Assata Shakur plays the dozens with Doblin.

Always the guiding light is the Black Freedom Movement. It is how to envision a future. America is buried under plastic and lies. We have to follow the North Star like our ancestors did before and stand on tippy-toes, pluck it from the sky, and place it on our tongue like a tab of LSD.

We have to read the night sky like a sheet of music.

We have to imagine freedoms that don't exist yet.

I wanted,
    I always wanted
I always wanted
    to return
to the body
    Where I was born

Allen Ginsberg, 1954

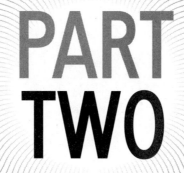

PART
TWO

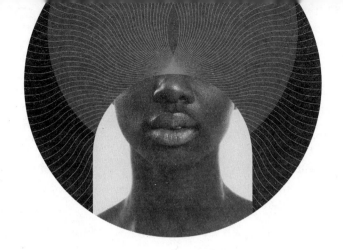

THE RETURN TO
THE BODY

"BROOKLYN, MAKE SOME NOISE!" THE DJ cupped his ear. "I can't hear you!" The crowd raised their hands and yelled. The bobbing faces leaned back in joy. Baritone yeses, laughter, and sharp falsetto howls echoed through Fort Greene Park. Soul Summit, the annual deep house dance-a-thon, was in full effect. A kaleidoscope of Black Brooklyn gathered for communion. The DJ was the priest. The beat was the Eucharist. We, the believers.

Wherever the eye turned was a portrait of Black joy. Sweat slicked, bare-chested brothers gyrated hips. Over there, a light sistah, reddish afro and freckles, was in a free-form salsa trance. Two Black gay men grinded and kissed. An elder in a dashiki sashayed from side to side on her cane. A tall West Indian man jumped, finger to the sky, and whipped his shirt like a propeller. We were packed tight, nearly skin-to-skin to share the hot summer sun and ride the hard, bone-bumping beat.

On the sidelines, couples and friends passed fat joints or vapes, clouds puffed like smoke signals, or sipped shots from brown-bagged liquor bottles. Many took Ecstasy or mushrooms. A few snorted snow.

Music and drugs took us to a higher place. Shimmering in the steam, almost touchable, was a vision of the homeland. Call it Zion. Call it Wakanda. Call it la Raza. The peak hit, and for a moment, everyone moved like a giant wave. We rose and fell and touched the ground again. The beat drove through us and drove out of us the lies we used to live and left us washed clean by sweat.

Stumbling off the dance floor, I kept looking back while walking away. In a pocket, I found a joint, half-smoked. Here, drugs were part of the ceremony.

Leaving Fort Greene Park, I saw the other side of drug use. On the church steps was a homeless drunk, passed out, urine darkening his pants. Fifteen minutes later, I turned on to my street; I sidestepped three addicts who made the corner their home, nodding off on heroin. Sitting on my stoop, I saw again in memory a night years ago, during a block party as children played, when an angry man who'd been drinking and smoking and picking fights left and came back with a gun, firing shots as we shielded the kids with our bodies.

Drugs heal. Drugs hurt. It is not the chemicals but the Set, Setting, and Container and its role in culture. At Soul Summit, weed, alcohol, and Ecstasy were a sacrament to a party that, for us, transcended hedonism and became spiritual. With each puff and swallow, we remembered how to love with fewer rules. No entry fees. No church dues. No Jesus. No Muhammad. No Moët on ice. No private club booths.

Walking home, I smiled at the hypocrisy. Every. Fucking. Day. We do "drugs." We gulp coffee by the gallon. In the morning, I see men blow steaming cups of joe as if kissing their reflections. We smoke cigarettes. We down Adderall like candy, an amphetamine—speed basically—to focus ADHD into the day's to-do list. In Bed-Stuy I can buy weed down the street, totally legit, but if I fly to Indiana and a cop sniffs weed in my car, I can be arrested. But across the border in Illinois, it's all good.

A drug spectrum exists. Imagine a one-to-ten scale, with one being legal and celebrated. The obvious on the lowest end is what I just said: coffee. At two to three, legal but not always cheered. Cigarettes definitely fall into this spot. Really up until the '90s a cigarette dangling in the mouth was a cool affectation. After the anti-smoking campaign, it looks dirty and cancerous. Four to six is not legal but also not a deal-breaker on a Tinder date. Like, hey, I did some Molly at a rave. Oh really, so did I! Made out with a gay best friend, I was so fucked up. Ha ha ha.

A little further up, things get dicey. Seven to eight, you might think twice about this person meeting your kids. Here lies powder cocaine or heroin. Nine and ten, users bear 666, the mark of the beast. Run, run as fast as you can! Meth, bath salts, and crack cocaine are right on the precipice; one step and you'll be "addicted" forever. The American storyline says if you do these drugs, you'll end up smoking crack while being sodomized by Nino Brown's Dobermans from *New Jack City*.

The drug spectrum goes from benign to fun, dangerous to disgusting. Each degree in the spectrum is an empty spot, and across history, one sees the same drug shifting like a game of musical chairs. Decades ago, alcohol was illegal. Remember the 1987 Brian De Palma film *The Untouchables*, set in the Prohibition era? Federal officer Eliot Ness, played by Kevin Costner, takes an axe to rum-filled barrels that Al Capone was smuggling into Chicago. Well, today A$AP Rocky buys billboards in downtown Brooklyn for his new whiskey Mercer + Prince. Take weed: When I was growing up in the '90s, it was illegal and subversive. Today marijuana stores do brisk business in New York and talk show hosts routinely yuk it up with actors or comedians like Seth Rogen or Bill Maher about smoking blunts.

For a long, long time, psychedelics, specifically LSD but also MDMA and mushrooms, were said to be gateways to madness. I fondly remember holding my first dose of LSD with butterflies in my stomach. Would it cause me to hallucinate bugs in my hair? Would I think I was a glass of orange juice, afraid of spilling? Would I lose my shit?

Today, psychedelics have been moved by a tidal wave of media from madness-inducing drugs to medicine. Books, TV, radio, podcasts, articles, celebrity testimonials, and films have repositioned MDMA and ketamine as cures. Peyote is a hands-off chemical because it is a tool of Indigenous ceremonies and the market demand led to overharvesting. Psilocybin (mushrooms) and LSD will be on the legalization conveyor belt. The term in activist circles is *psychedelic exceptionalism* because they are now separated from the criminal-addiction story of the other "bad drugs." They are exempt from drug stigma. What bothers the hell out of a lot of my friends is the background racism. Psychedelics are linked to white people, mostly Hippie, festival, club-going, rave-hopping whites who come off as goofy, nice kids. The association to whiteness washes them of criminality.

Slowly the story of psychedelics is changing in our Communities of Color. The actual use of LSD, mushrooms, or MDMA, much less Indigenous plant medicines like peyote or ayahuasca, is very, very low among us. As more testimonials come out, the needle moves. The question remains as to what it would take for psychedelics to be a part of the drug use by People of Color? How does it play a role in our liberation?

I ask that a lot and sometimes the answer is to laugh at myself. While walking home from Soul Summit, I tried to shoehorn psychedelics into our lives. I saw a brother sporting a fresh face and a Vans T-shirt, lopsided from shouldering a laptop. He waved to the Yemeni bodega deli man, who smoked a cigarette and wiped hands on his apron while smiling at the post office worker, who brought mail and moved out of the way of three white women in Gucci shades, hurrying into a pottery class. It struck me as just ever so slightly crazy to be like, "Hey, folks, here's some acid. I promise it will unveil a world of beauty that far surpasses this mundane, cruel one we endure. Wanna try a hit?"

Psychedelics may be now an "exception" but in terms of use, overall, minuscule. They lag far behind getting drunk on Friday night or getting high on Saturday at the club. To be a political force, they need to connect to healing in a way the masses can embrace. Which means accessible psychedelics and free or affordable therapy may be covered by Medicare or Medicaid or private insurance and group circles to integrate personal healing into the larger community. Also we need a clear explanation of what the therapy part of psychedelic therapy is. One place to find it is in our history and literature.

What makes drugs—whether ingested, snorted, smoked, or swallowed—a therapeutic experience is their *role in Transference.* When I got home from Soul Summit, I perused my bookshelves and pulled out the 1973 book *The Language of Psycho-Analysis* by Jean Laplanche and Jean Bertrand Pontalis, two French theorists who refined Sigmund Freud's work. I read the entry on Transference: "Actualisation of unconscious wishes . . . infantile prototypes re-emerge and are experienced with a strong sensation of immediacy" (455). Fingering the page, I studied the line, "Freud stresses that it is connected with 'prototypes' or imagos (chiefly the imago of the father, but also of the mother, brother, etc.): the doctor is inserted 'into one of the psychical "series" which the patient has already formed,'" and further down, "Transference on to the person of the physician is triggered off precisely at the moment when particularly important repressed contents are in danger of being revealed" (458). At the end I had highlighted, "Transference becomes the terrain upon which the patient's unique set of problems is played out with an ineluctable immediacy, the area where the subject finds himself face-to-face with the existence, the permanence and the force of his unconscious wishes and phantasies: 'It is on that field that the victory must be won'" (458). I tapped my finger on those sentences that were like a string of pearls.

Closing my eyes, I remembered my experience in therapy. I sat in a comfy room as the therapist placed questions on me like suction tubes. She barely blinked, which unnerved me. The more I talked, the less I was aware of her, and I relived an old conflict. I hashed it out with Mom or Dad, a friend or lover. Tears burned. Finally I said what I needed to. It felt like coughing up lightning. The spell snapped. I was back in the here and now. My therapist gently smiled; good work had been done. Transference.

I slid a book from the shelf and smelled its pages. A rustic musk like an old man's hair rose from it. The title was *LSD Psychotherapy: An Exploration of Psychedelic and Psycholytic Therapy* by W. V. Caldwell, published in 1968, the peak of the Hippie acid movement. He traveled to clinics in England and America where patients were treated with LSD. They wrestled their unconscious like fighters in a steel cage match; it was powerful writing. He, too, talked about the role of Transference:

> Transference is, if anything, a more useful tool in psychedelic therapy, for the process is more active and hence more easily observed and analyzed. Here it is not difficult to achieve a transference; it is almost impossible to avoid it. Some petty frustration sets off a boiling rage at the therapist. The patient bellows and fumes—and in the middle of a sentence he sees his father's face before him in a similar childhood

situation. Suddenly he knows why he is angry. Shortly after he may recall a series of annoyances stretching back through time and discovers all these piques were but escape valves for the original hatred buried in his mind. (71)

Closing the book, I felt again Soul Summit's pounding 120 beats per minute. Weed, drink, and MDMA melted the "I" into gyrating hips and popping feet. I felt the "unconscious wish" to be one with the People, mi Gente, pulled up from crotch to navel, chest to mouth, and I shouted, "Yooooo!" My Transference "prototype" or "imago" was not a singular parental figure as in Freud's definition but the *whole family*.

At Soul Summit, dance *was* the doctor. The ancestors we paid homage to were, in a sense, watching us, and we watched ourselves through them. The more we spun, drank, and smoked, the closer we came to a truth we repressed in our lives. We want revolutionary joy to redeem us from the nightmare of whiteness.

I wish I could say it's just me, but it's not. In our minds is a toxic brew of internalized racism, classism, sexism, and homophobia. Dammit if we don't visit it upon each other in brutal and intimate ways. Especially if it's the hood. We fear that when we pull up, be it the stoop or club, or waiting in line or at the bar, that we'll be hurt, embarrassed, or hustled by our own kind. Just let someone step on a homie's sneakers or hit on his girl and a gun will be pulled. I woke up to so many gunshots outside my window. Neighbors showed me bullet scars. On more intimate levels, it is there too. On dates, we tense up at colorist jokes. If we are gay, we tiptoe on eggshells around brothers on the corner who always have some fucking bullshit to say.

Yet in those bejeweled moments at Soul Summit, we get a glimpse of what a new world could be. We pull up in cowrie shells, Puerto Rican flags, Malcolm X hats, turbans, and African pendants; we are saying, "Not today, Satan!" This dance is not just for us, it's for our ancestors—Taínos, Yorubas, Arawaks, Fulani—who couldn't dance in chains. When we slap hands, say "brother" and "sister" and "fam," joy explodes the eyes; it's us seeing us as if for the first time, reborn like babies, and the infantile prototypes come surging back in as we reconnect with our family, our history, ourselves. Transference? Yes, but something beyond it, more powerful and traditional. Collective Transference.

But where did I hear this before? Where did I read about Collective Transference? I pulled *The Autobiography of Malcolm X* from the shelf, found a bookmark in chapter four titled "Laura" and read:

> I still harbored one secret humiliation: I couldn't dance. I can't remember when it was that I actually learned how . . . But dancing was the chief action at those "pad parties," . . . With alcohol or marijuana lightening my head, and that wild music wailing away on those portable record players, it didn't take long to loosen up the dancing instincts in my African heritage . . . I was up in the jostling crowd—and suddenly, unexpectedly, I got the idea. It was as though somebody had clicked on a light. My long-suppressed African instincts broke through, and loose. (59–60)

Malcolm X wrote that scene, but Malcolm Little lived it. Standing to the side, he nursed his secret shame until "some girl grabbed [him]," and swoosh! Swept up in music, high and buzzed, Malcolm X returned to his body. To do so he had to break through years of internalized racism:

> Having spent so much time in Mason's white environment, I had always believed and feared that dancing involved a certain order or pattern of specific steps—as dancing is done by whites. But here among my own less inhibited people, I discovered it was simply letting your feet, hands and body spontaneously act out whatever impulses were stirred by the music. (60)

Music . . . and drugs. Classic cocktail. Malcom X was clear on how the "alcohol or marijuana lightening my head," or in other words, dissolved the superego, the part of the psyche that Laplanche and Pontalis defined as "one of the agencies of the personality . . . the super-ego's role in relation to the ego may be compared to that of a judge or censor" (435). Malcolm X was "judging" and "censoring" himself from the viewpoint of the whites he grew up with, and in a sense, they grew inside him and formed part of his ego.

For us, racial minorities in the United States, the superego is also a *white* superego. We are born into a white power structure. The faces of authority and privilege, in our classrooms or state capitals, titans of business or elite celebrities, are often *white*. The scales on which we will be measured are *white*. It creates a white superego floating like a military satellite spying on you from space. We watch ourselves. We police ourselves. We carefully monitor how we think and act and feel.

Not all the time. We don't whip ourselves with the American flag like some medieval flagellant during the plague. Malcolm was nuanced. He notes how some whites were cool. He was chill. Not at zero but not cranked to ten either. Racist whites? He was keyed up. In those scenes, Malcolm X was hyperaware of the white superego and the life-and-death risks that could spring like a trap in an Indiana Jones movie. One misstep and some Founding Father's head, like a giant boulder, would roll over him.

The role of drugs in *The Autobiography of Malcolm X* was to dissolve the white superego. As it disintegrates, the body reemerges. Malcolm returned to his body and listened to its pulsing joys; the music plucked nerves as if he were a giant guitar. His feet snapped in time as he instantaneously read his dance partner's moves and matched them in effortless flow. When he writes, "long-suppressed African instincts" were freed, it's over-the-top. People all over the world, from Dublin to Hong Kong, dance with abandon. It's not an "African" thing.

What is important is he codes his body's truth as "African," so when he returns to it, he returns to his people, who he had been separated from by the white superego. As much as his transformation from Malcolm Little to Malcolm X is seen as the result of tutelage in Islam and Black Nationalism by Elijah Muhammad's Nation of Islam, the reality is that his first rediscovery of Blackness came through getting turned up. It was at this alcohol- and weed-filled party that his metamorphosis happened.

The Return to the Body is the key concept of the Black diaspora. When Black people reembrace the body, relish kinky hair and skin hues from brown to beige, toffee to obsidian, revel in it, squeeze from it deep pain and pleasure, a nuclear blast of energy is released that transports one to *a psychedelic state*. It fuels the forward motion into new Black consciousness, one that envisions the end of this cruel racist nation and the start of a new one. Which is why, reading the Black Literary Canon, one can trace this powerful nostalgia. In the mountain of books by Black authors, activists, and leaders, the Return to the Body is a bright vein of Pan-African gold.

Thirty-six years before *The Autobiography of Malcolm X* was published, Black author Zora Neale Hurston published in 1928 an essay titled, "How It Feels to Be Colored Me" in the journal *The World Tomorrow*. In it, again, the Black author writes a head-spinning story about music and joy and ancestor worship in language that evokes synesthesia. Hurston retells an experience at a jazz club:

> For instance, when I sit in the drafty basement that is the New World Cabaret with a white person, my color comes. We enter chatting about any little nothing that we have in common and are seated by the jazz waiters. In the abrupt way that jazz orchestras have, this one plunges into a number. It loses no time in circumlocutions but gets right down to business. It constricts the thorax and splits the heart with its tempo and narcotic harmonies. This orchestra grows

rambunctious, rears on its hind legs and attacks the tonal veil with primitive fury, rending it, clawing it until it breaks through to the jungle beyond. I follow those heathen—follow them exultingly. I dance wildly inside myself; I yell within, I whoop; I shake my assegai above my head, I hurl it true to the mark yeeeeooww! I am in the jungle and living in the jungle way. My face is painted red and yellow, and my body is painted blue, My pulse is throbbing like a war drum. I want to slaughter something—give pain, give death to what, I do not know. But the piece ends. The men of the orchestra wipe their lips and rest their fingers. I creep back slowly to the veneer we call civilization with the last tone and find the white friend sitting motionless in his seat smoking calmly.

"Good music they have here," he remarks, drumming the table with his fingertips.

Music. The great blobs of purple and red emotion have not touched him. He has only heard what I felt. He is far away and I see him but dimly across the ocean and the continent that have fallen between us. He is so pale with his whiteness then and I am so colored. (1032)

Again, the Return to the Body. Again, the recycled racial tropes of African primitivism that were standard white supremacy, but reversing them, Hurston exposed the buried body and released it. Malcolm called it "African instincts." Hurston calls it "the jungle way." Neither are accurate. It is Transference, where the prototype or image of a free African ancestor functions as the blank surface to project desire. The image of the preslavery African (even if a historical fiction) was a way to express rage at white supremacy and bypass internalized racism. When she writes, "My pulse is throbbing like a war drum. I want to slaughter something—give pain, give death to what, I do not know," it's clear from the line, "with a white person, my color comes," Hurston is "slaughtering" her own *white* superego.

The Return to the Body through Collective Transference works in a series of identifiable stages and interlocking various elements. First is the heady thrill of submersion in the ocean of others, the ecstasy of being one drop in a flowing river of people. Snatching Sigmund Freud's 1921 book *Group Psychology and the Analysis of the Ego* from the shelf, I read that "in a group the individual is brought under conditions which allow him to throw off the repressions of his unconscious instincts" (666). Second, the body does in public what the patient's speech does in therapy: it undergoes free association. It moves. It grooves. It reenacts. Desires repressed by the white superego rise to the surface and are pulled magnetically by the imago or prototype of a parental figure; at times it is the ancestors who are conjured, whether in symbols worn (cowrie shells, Boricua T-shirt), a leader's presence (Rev. Al Sharpton, a Santería priestess), or ceremony (Middle Passage offering, BLM protests) or anniversary. Overwhelming the white superego by this Collective Transference is signaled by joyful euphoria, an intense psychedelic "oceanic" perspective of oneness, often followed by synesthesia and creativity. The Return to the Body heals us and rejuvenates Black consciousness. The "I" flows into the immense river of birth and death, cleansed of shame, fear, or pettiness by realizing it is a mere drop in an eternal force.

It is important to note that elements can be present but not combine into Collective Transference. In Hurston's 1934 essay "Characteristics of Negro Expressions" where she talks of Southern jook joints, she said, "Jook is the word for Negro pleasure house. It may mean a bawdy house. It may mean the house set apart on public works where men and women dance, drink and gamble" (1049). She described the barely held together shacks of the Black Belt, trash-filled yards where folks gulped down gut-wrenching moonshine. Yes, the drugs and drink and dancing are present. Missing is the link to the larger history, the Transference to the ancestors, and the healing of the people.

Closer to Collective Transference are the Vodou dances in the West Indies, where a priest or priestess pounds a drum as devotees are "possessed" by Shango, Ogun, or Yemeya. Entering a trance, the dancer is gripped like a rag doll by the immense power of a god. Limbs spasm as if by supernatural voltage. Missing is the political dimension that commits one to action in the here and now. Otherwise, it becomes religious escapism.

The Return to the Body that leads to a Collective Transference has been and remains a key dynamic of the Black diaspora. One sees it in the past. Native peoples and enslaved Africans scooped up the shards of cultures that survived European genocide and the Middle Passage. Old songs were sung in the master's language. Old gods worshipped in secret. Old ways passed down in fables and myths.

It is odd to look through enslaver records and see how furiously people fought to feel. On plantations when the sun dipped and work ended, or at a funeral or Sundays at Congo Square in Louisiana, enslaved Black people shook off chains and then the very memory of chains. In John W. Blassingame's 1972 book, *The Slave Community*, he cited a Southern white who described Black dancing: "Clapping hands was their music and distorting their frames into the most unnatural figures and emitting hideous noises . . . " (39). One can see rage and trauma jetting from limbs like a fire hose.

I put the books back and see embedded in the whole library flashing scenes of Collective Transference. You see it in works from Frederick Douglass's 1845 slave narrative to W. E. B. Du Bois's 1935 *Black Reconstruction in America* to Sapphire's 1996 novel, *Push*. I could just close my eyes, pluck a book out, and with enough time, be sure that here it was again.

Here was the truth. Transference or the "actualization of unconscious wishes" is for the oppressed innately political. In modern therapy, in a clinic with a psychodynamic therapist trained in one of the Freudian branches, free association eases the superego. The pressurized memories and emotions surge to the surface and projected onto the therapist. When the patient is a Person of Color, not all of the material, but a lot, is connected to how much racism walled them off from themselves. A catalog of symptoms, projections, introjections, complexes, traumas, and Double-Consciousness are congealed like gooey Jell-O in the brain. A deep curing transformation takes place, like a butterfly emerging from a chrysalis. Who knows that when a butterfly flaps its wings, it causes a hurricane to spin across the world?

Here was another truth. In the Black Literary Canon, Collective Transference does not occur in a therapist's office. Black, Latino, Asian, and Indigenous people had little access to therapy. Even less to the psychedelic therapy that was briefly legal that W. V. Caldwell wrote about in his *LSD Psychotherapy*. Transference was not channeled through the Medical Model but through community; Transference rocked streets in both party or protest. Malcolm X and Hurston describing the joy of rediscovering their bodies at a club were minuscule portraits of a larger dynamic. When the lens is pulled back, what happened to them happens to millions who are an immense river of consciousness breaking through the dam to irrigate the body. It is a power that sweeps whole peoples in its currents. So far, in these two examples, we only glimpsed this titanic force as if peering through a peephole.

After looking at the Black Literary Canon, we can already see the promise of psychedelic therapy is betrayed by the Medical Model. Yes, it will succeed in making it legal. Yes, a therapist will place a pill in your palm. The doctor's office will be clean and comfy. You can lie on a bed or couch. Scented candles will perfume the room. A glowing crystal and music will create a relaxed vibe. Yes, you can dive deep into yourself, the pressure increases, and you will be tossed and thrown by memories and wrestle with versions of you, clawing like monsters in the dark. All of this is needed work. All of this cures.

Leaving the therapist's office, you will have a small healing. One that fits in your hands. Outside in the world it must be protected, like holding a candle flame close so the wind doesn't blow it out.

If that is the extent of psychedelic therapy, then the true meaning of Transference will be lost. What we experience, what we see, what we project on the therapists is a montage of archaic pain trapped inside us. If we look through it as if holding up a lens, our pain teaches us to see why others suffer. How it repeats across our separate lives because it is stamped into our bodies by the same systems as being trapped on a conveyor belt in a demonic factory where soft flesh is pulped and hammered by steel pins. Call it patriarchy. Call it capitalism. Call it white supremacy. Call it by its many names. Call it out.

Standing on tiptoes, I got a joint from the cupboard and lit it. Malcolm X's book was on the desk. I reread the scene of him drinking and smoking weed at the party. How he loosened his body and danced like there's no tomorrow. Tall ass Malcolm, gangly legs and arms, spinning and sliding and bobbing on the balls of his feet. I could see him buzzing, the weed smoke erasing the "self" as the drink burned in the belly.

"Here's to you, Malcolm." I inhaled, coughed, inhaled more.

Powerful as it is to read drugs as liberation, I had to be real about it. Very few scenes in the Black Literary Canon positioned drugs of any kind as a pathway to freedom. The Return to the Body that I saw in Malcolm X and Zora Neale Hurston that involved at least alcohol and, in Malcolm's case, weed was incredibly rare.

What they showed me was how important Transference was in fighting internalized racism. I had a suspicion that the Return to the

Body and Collective Transference were not just in personal stories. No, it was larger than that. It was world-shattering.

I took down from the shelf Caribbean historian C. L. R. James's classic study of the 1791 Haitian Revolution, the 1938 book *The Black Jacobins*. I saw in it a world-historical Collective Transference that wrecked slavery and set in motion a grinding, halting, breakdown of global white supremacy. As I read, his words were a paintbrush held by an Expressionist, using bright strokes of color to bring the past to life.

Haiti was a pressure cooker. Under a punishing sun, wealthy white enslavers sat on top of poor whites who oversaw enslaved Africans. They worked them from sunup to sundown. They worked them to the breaking point, really to the edge of death. Some fled, and those who were caught were whipped until skin hung from bone like rags or were tied to a post and burned alive in public to crispy meat.

The immense weight of the powerful wore the people down to the primal instinct to live. James described the spark of Haiti's revolution. Dutty Boukman, a runaway from Jamaica, told a gathering of Haitians it was time to seize the moment. A storm lashed the island like a giant claw of wind and water. It was for many a sign. They must *be the storm*. Boukman said, "The God who is so good orders us to vengeance. He will direct our hands and give us help. Throw away the image of the God of the whites who thirst for our tears. Listen to the liberty that speaks in all our hearts" (87). A Vodou priestess named Cécile Fatiman was possessed by the loas and danced and cut the throat of a pig. Sharing its blood with the Haitians, she told them to kill the slaveowners on the island.

See the elements of a Collective Transference, the group psychology opening a path for repressed desire. The projection onto a parental figure, in this case, God. The overcoming of the internalized white superego and a Return to the Body. See the dancing. See the psychedelic state of embracing or integrating one's fragmented and suppressed consciousness into a whole one. See the revolution from being trapped in the master's authority and revolving back to your own body. See blood as the lubricant.

A fever forced me to search the shelf. I plucked W. E. B. Du Bois's *Black Reconstruction*, and sure enough, here it is, the second scene of Collective Transference that changed world history. It was the Emancipation Proclamation.

Slave revolts had exploded in the South, the Caribbean, and tip to tip of the Americas. In the 1943 book *American Negro Slave Revolts*, author Herbert Aptheker found evidence of two hundred and fifty rebellions in the antebellum US, from as small as a dozen to the platoon size of Nat Turner's 1831 revolt. Turner led a lightning charge of slaves wielding knives and blunt tools to smash the skulls of slaveowners. Uprisings spiked in the US, and the Civil War broke out. Canons spat fire. Union and Confederate soldiers thrust bayonets into bellies and shot and shot and shot. Bloated corpses filled the land like human-sized water balloons.

In the end, Black Americans could not wage revolution. They were a minority. Haitians, a majority. Yet they pulled the one lever they had, which was their labor. Du Bois wrote of a general strike by Black enslaved workers: "The trickling streams of fugitives swelled to a flood. Once, begun the general strike of black and white went madly and relentlessly on like some great saga" (64). Trodding on dirt roads, thousands of Black families left the South. They brought down its economy and, therefore, its ability to wage a war meant to keep them enslaved.

Du Bois wrote the most enduring description of Collective Transference. He dove into the archive and uncovered the truth: Black America experienced a once-in-a-millennium, titanic, soul-shattering Collective Transference. He wrote, "But to most of the four million black folk emancipated by civil war, God was real. They knew Him. They had met Him personally in many a wild orgy of religious frenzy, or in the black stillness of night. His plan for them was clear; they were to suffer and be degraded, and then afterwards by Divine edict, raised to manhood and power; and so . . . He made them free" (124). Later he added a more powerful endnote:

> It was all foolish, bizarre and tawdry. Gangs of dirty Negroes howl-ing and dancing; poverty stricken ignorant laborers mistaking war, destruction and revolution for the mystery of the free human soul; and yet to these black folk it was Apocalypse. The magnificent trumpet tones of Hebrew scripture, transmuted and oddly changed became a strange new Gospel. All that was Beauty. All that was love, all that was Truth, stood on top of these mad mornings and sang with the stars. A great human sob shrieked in the wind, and tossed its tears upon the sea—free, free, free.

> There was joy in the South. It rose like perfume—like a prayer. Men stood quivering. Slim dark girls, wild and beautiful with wrinkled hair, wept silently; young women, black, tawny, white and golden, lifted shivering hands, and old and broken mothers, black and gray, raised great voice and shouted to God across the field and up to the rocks and the mountains. (124)

Again, the elements of Collective Transference. Group psychol-ogy that, as Freud said, allows the one to "throw off the repressions of his unconscious instincts." Again, projection onto a parental author-ity, here it's the God of Exodus to bypass the white superego. The euphoric Return to the Body in the "great human sob" and the people who "shouted to God." In this euphoric psychedelic state, the veil is torn and a new world born.

Imagine being there at the birth of a new freedom. Imagine a man hesitantly poking his head out of a slave cabin and hearing rumors of emancipation. He sees on the road war refugees heading to the Union Army, his friends, his family, bewildered and tired but guided by a holy vision. He had been a scared man, all his life flinching at the cracking whips, a man who kept his eyes low to avoid beatings. Now his heart kicked in his chest like a horse. A terrible, beautiful force pushed his feet across the doorway. He walked, ran, sprinted. Aunts yelled for him, but he ran like the wind. Brothers and sisters tackled and held him down, fanned his face, wiped tears, and said over and over, "Breathe. Breathe."

Lifetimes of trauma, whipped, beaten, and raped into Black bodies erupted like a volcano. Lava hot dreams flowed into song and prayer. In that euphoria, a path to freedom became visible. It is a centuries-long path that one may not live to see, but you knew one day, great-great-great grandchildren you could never touch would find it.

Heavy stuff. Putting *Black Reconstruction* down, I realized I was breathing fast. Here was proof that the idea existed. Collective Transference is the mighty wheel that spun whole epochs and governments upside down. It takes an alienated consciousness and returns it to the body. It frees the masses to flow to their power.

Seeing through this concept, the questions around psychedelics shift. Really of drugs in general. It is not if they are legal or illegal. It is not about chemical composition or the interaction with the brain. It is what their role is in igniting Personal and Collective Transference that leads to an integration of the repressed desire for freedom.

Sliding Du Bois back on the shelf, I looked at the books and saw the Return to the Body like a vein of gold glittering in rock. Here are petrified voices of ancestors: Assata Shakur and Frederick Douglass, Ntozake Shange and Piri Thomas. Touching titles, I remembered where they rediscovered themselves. The words throbbed on the page as if pulsing with life.

In my own life, I experienced Collective Transference. During the 2008 presidential campaign, a little-known Black senator from Chicago named Barack Obama ran for the White House. He seemed like a nod to diversity but nothing to pin our hopes on. Yet wherever he went, huge crowds, *white* crowds magnetized. A strange electricity surrounded him. Long-suppressed hope shot from the belly and illuminated him. Obama acknowledged this effect in his 2006 book, *Audacity of Hope*, saying, "I serve as a blank screen on which people of vastly different political stripes project their own views" (34). What we projected, or more accurately, what we transferred onto him, was the hope that King's dream of entering the promised land would come true. He was our Joshua.

When Obama won, I remember the ground-shaking street parties from Brooklyn to Harlem. We danced. I took Ecstasy. Floating on joy, we felt that night that America had embraced our full selves. We could be Black and Latino and Asian and Native *and* American. We screamed and drank as police looked on, sometimes smiling and dancing with us. We sang the national anthem. We waved the flag.

Looking back, none of us predicted it would be the beginning of a brutal white backlash, a reactionary turn to Nazism that culminated in the election of Donald Trump. It was a halcyon once-in-a-century celebration, our Collective Transference. For one night, early in the twenty-first century, we returned to ourselves.

≩ ≩ ≩

Taking Cross's "The Negro-to-Black Conversion Experience," I hold the essay up to the bookshelves like a treasure map to a bright light. Squinting, I saw the Return to the Body glow like a secret ideogram between stages. I reread the Pre-Encounter; Cross defined it as the time we are, "programmed to think the world as being non-Black, anti-Black, or the opposite of Black. The person's worldview is dominated by the Euro-American determinants" (15). Moving down to the next step, the Encounter, I scrupulously read:

> The Encounter is a verbal or visual event . . . for example, the death of Martin Luther King Jr. hurled thousands of pre-encounter Negroes into a search for a deeper understanding of the Black Power Movement. Witnessing a friend being assaulted by the police, televised reports of racial incidents, or discussions with a friend or loved one who is further advanced into his own Blackness may 'turn a person on' to his own Blackness. (17)

For Cross, Moral Shock recoils one from white supremacy. Horrific violence does it. God knows we have got enough of that in America. It forces a visceral disgust of racism and to dig deeper; it demands one reckon with our complicity. Cross foretold a dynamic that sociologist James Jasper coined twenty-six years later in his 1997 book, *The Art of Moral Protest*, as a Moral Shock. He defined it as "an unexpected event or piece of information which raises such a sense of outrage in a person that she becomes inclined toward political action" (39). Moral Shock makes visible two sets of opposing values grinding one against the other until the social hypocrisy is exposed like a bloody fingernail scratch.

Cross cited the 1968 assassination of King. He was a Christian pastor, shot in cold blood for advocating peace. Moral Shock. Riots.

In 1955, Emmett Till was a fourteen-year-old boy, falsely accused of wolf-whistling a white woman. White racists blew his brains out. The innocence of a child desecrated by violence. Moral Shock. A reenergized Civil Rights Movement.

In our own time, George Floyd was choked to death by officer Derek Chauvin, who kneeled on his neck for nine minutes, smirking as bystanders begged him to stop. Floyd cried for his mom. Moral Shock. Nearly twenty-six million joined BLM marches that shook America and the world.

Moral Shock is one ignition of a Return to the Body because it forces the oppressed to resee the horror of the system. Rage burns away authority and its symbols. Rage pushes aside the ruling class–based superego. When the cop, the priest, the president, the teacher, the judge, the boss are finally out of your head, you stand and look at calloused hands and feel, maybe for the first time, the shortness of breath, the weight of the fear and hurt carried in muscle. You come back to your body, cleansed of hope. You realize you lied to yourself. You truly hoped that if you followed rules, you'd be safe. But you never were.

Yet looking through Cross's essay back to the Black voices sandwiched on the shelf, seeing Du Bois, seeing Assata, seeing Audre Lorde, it was clear that Moral Shock led to a social movement *only* under very precise conductions. First, power dynamics had to shift and make a fissure through which Black folks could dismantle part of white supremacy. In *The Black Jacobins*, James drew a vivid portrait of enslavers vastly outnumbered by the enslaved, seething and watching for a time to strike. In *Black Reconstruction*, Du Bois showed Black people leaving Southern plantations in the fog of war to cripple the economy. Black life in a white supremacy is always in a war of maneuver, angling for leverage.

The other way, I could see right in front of me. Pulling Assata Shakur's autobiography, Lynne Fauley Emery's *Black Dance: From 1619 to Today*, and Amiri Baraka's *The LeRoi Jones / Amiri Baraka Reader*; you see love, relentless love is the other ignition for the Return to the Body. See it in our joy. See it in our pleasure. See it in our communion. In church, sparks lead to a mysterious alchemy. The congregation "catch the spirit." Look at the gay ballroom dances in *Paris Is Burning*. They catch the spirit too. Go to a BLM or Occupy Wall Street rally and feel the festival atmosphere. Hugs, dance, and laughter warm the air. In DC on Juneteenth, folks cut loose and feel free. And yes, you see it in deep house events like Soul Summit, where heartbeats race to catch the 120 beats per minute. Love is an ignition for the Return to the Body. It is not based on a reaction to the violence of white supremacy or what Jasper called a Moral Shock. Which is *reactive*. Which is unsustainable. Only a movement based on ever-expanding love can last because love feeds us. Love builds. Love heals. Love is the promised land.

Going back to Cross's essay, I put my finger on the Immersion-Emersion stage. Here it was that the body radiates like a secret on a yellowed treasure map. Cross says, "The person immerses himself in the world of Blackness" and "Immersion is a strong powerful dominating sensation constantly being energized by Black rage, guilt, a third and new fuel, a developing sense of pride. As one brother put it, 'I was swept along by a sea of Blackness'" (18). In one beautiful description, Cross collects the raw change he witnessed in his friends, his family, and himself. Imagine a domino effect of white masks falling from face after face, on the ground like ceramic bowls breaking to pieces.

> Everything that is Black is good and romantic. The person accepts his hair, his brown skin is "beautiful." That a person exists and is Black is an inherently wonderful phenomenon . . . One spends a great deal of time developing an Afro hair style, and it becomes more common to wear African-inspired clothing . . . During the immersion-emersion stage the person has a creative burst . . . people who never before sought or experienced creative activity discover they are able to express themselves in a totally new mode. (18)

The Return to the Body is here. When the brotha said, "I was swept along by a sea of Blackness," one can track the group psychology that liberates the unconscious. Second, desire repressed by the white superego is pulled magnetically by the imago or prototype of a parental figure. Cross cited King's murder as the slaying of a "father" or the Moses of the people. Fuck if we don't feel that all the time. I think of George Floyd as our collective "uncle" or Trayvon Martin as our collective "little brother" or "son."

It is followed by joy. I remembered what Hurston imagined, the "pure African" as in the ancestors who were once free, conjured in today's afros, dashikis, and BLM protests. Step shows too. The overwhelming of the white superego by Collective Transference comes with joyful euphoria, a Return to the Body in an explosion that Cross says is expressed as a "burst of creativity."

The books, Cross's essay, my own life, the stories others told me—all of these pieces fit together into a coherent theory. Under the tornado of thoughts spinning in our skulls, the body pulsed in profane innocence. It hungers. It thirsts. It knows. It feels. It wants to speak its true name aloud.

It made me wonder. Who else is trapped? If there is a "Negro-to-Black Conversion Experience" is there also a "Woman-to-Feminist" or "Closeted-to-Gay" or "Worker-to-Proletariat" conversion?

Is this a theory that can explain the past? Predict the future? What does this say about the political and cultural frames for therapy and psychedelic therapy in particular? Do the models we have of individual therapy in a legal setting betray the world-historical forces in the unconscious and what forms would set it free?

First, I blinked and followed that Return of the Body glowing like liquid gold, splitting into rivulets, dripping down the spines of books in nearby shelves. So many of us, alive here and now or those long faded to dust, experienced this joy.

Maybe psychedelics can shift gears in the Return of the Body from one ignited by Moral Shock to one sparked by Prophetic Love. Imagine a revolution sparked by wonder, awe, and the sublime? There would be no speed limit. No end to how far.

What if psychedelic therapy was leveled up from one-on-one visits in an office to cultural ceremonies in Madison Square Garden, the African Burial Ground, Central Park, Prospect Park, Coney Island Beach, the Rockaways? What if psychedelics were given like the holy wafer at Holy Communion? What if we ran headfirst into trauma, seeing it as the key to freeing our minds?

To begin imagining it, we first have to ask, What does the Return to the Body look like beyond the African diaspora?

What of the worker?

Every day, we work. In the turquoise dawn, trucks clang on the streets as garbage men haul trash. We work. Bodega shutters rattle up. Commuters drive long drives. We work. Children are dressed and dropped off at school. We work. We clean trains and wash laundry. We cook for restaurants. Steam mixes with sweat. We teach kids. We fix fiber optic cables. We write reports. We repair engines. We work.

And I know, many, maybe most of us, feel we lose something in work we can't get back. Not just time. Not just health. We lose our freedom to choose what to do and who to be. What money we earn can't pay for feeling smaller and smaller when we walk through the front door at home.

Plucking *The Visual History of the World* from the shelf, I turned its pages like a flipbook, where you see the image move as a cartoon. Here was the worker, an eternal figure through centuries, face dripping with sweat. They swung a sickle at tall wheat grass in the Neolithic era. In this chapter, they carried trays of food in ancient Rome. In the next one, they pulled levers of a mighty steam factory in England.

They, too, fought to return to their bodies. They, too, waited for a power shift, eyed when the position of their masters weakened.

They, too, called to whatever god or gods they prayed to for deliverance. The decision to strike seemed to come from a depth inside their bodies, a place of such high pressure that words were crushed into instinct.

It is, again, so incredibly odd to read the ruling class give voice to the voiceless, in effect testify for those they exploited and feared. I picked up a book on Spartacus and read a Roman official named Diodorus Siculus. I can feel Siculus's hand tremble writing about the First Servile War, "A large number of slaves joined the rebels. The slaves first inflicted extreme savageries on their own masters, and then turned to slaughter the rest of the inhabitants" (83). Repeatedly in history, the corpses of masters are the stepping-stones the oppressed use to climb back into their own bodies.

Nearly two thousand years after Siculus wrote of the slave rebellion, German Romantic philosopher Georg Wilhelm Hegel wrote in his 1807 book, *The Phenomenology of Spirit,* a section titled "Lordship and Bondage." It is one of the most important passages in Western philosophy. It eerily parallels Cross's "Negro-to-Black Conversion Experience" essay that came 164 years later. I held Hegel's book and Cross's essay in my hands as if on a weighing scale, amazed at how they balanced on the same idea: How does a consciousness, alienated outside of its body, return to its fully lived being?

Hegel, like Cross, came of age during a revolution. Imagine getting into a time machine and being whisked through a rip in space-time, almost like falling through a kaleidoscope tube and popping out in eighteenth-century Germany. Walking on the street is a young man with wide eyes, a big nose like a shark's fin, and pit bull–like jowls. He carries books and a rolled newspaper under his armpit. You watch him lean on a wall, thumbing pages. Hegel read everything, everywhere, all the time. He churned books in his mind like a grain mill, mulching the ideas into a vision of an ever-roving World Spirit, like a flame that traveled from one civilization to the next, growing hotter as humanity progressed toward Absolute Freedom. At nineteen, long before he wrote systemic philosophy, Hegel felt this World Spirit embodied in the French Revolution.

Imagine again, Hegel ambling along a cobblestone street, newspaper rolled in his fist, waving excitedly to schoolmates. Playfully he thumped them with it; they rushed to a pub, drank foamy beer, and read news of French revolutionaries storming the Bastille. Here was the World Spirit Hegel had imagined, now in reality, consuming all in its path.

Like Cross, inspired by the 1968 rebellions, Hegel was swept up in the 1789 upheaval, high on giddy hope of a new world. In 1807, he distilled that radicalism into the section in *The Phenomenology of Spirit* about the lord and the bondsman, where two beings engage in a fight for recognition.

Opening the book is an act of communion with countless readers who parsed this passage for clues on how to decipher their own epochs. Philosophers Martin Heidegger, Karl Marx, Martin Luther King Jr., Jean-Paul Sartre, Alexandre Kojève, Angela Davis, Amiri Baraka, Cedric Robinson, and Cornel West. Instantly you see why. It moves you in an uncomfortable yet familiar way. Almost like reading a horoscope, it's vague enough to see yourself in it. And in this edition, the font is old and the paper has a whiff of dust and time.

In "Lordship and Bondage," a battle begins like in every Hollywood film you've seen; maybe Russell Crowe in *Gladiator* or Sam Worthington and Stephen Lang in the *Avatar* films. The opponents try to wrest recognition from each other. In Hegel's prose, in the contest for power, one "comes out of itself" but immediately is "lost in the other" and has to find a way to "return unto itself" (111). In the "life-and-death struggle," the loser becomes a bondsman to the victor, who now is a lord that commands the bondsman, a "dependent consciousness" that sets aside its own desires, its own will in order to obey the lord.

Okay, simple enough. Sounds like a hyped-up playground fight. The bondsman labors for the lord, making on command, filling the world with objects. With each action, the bondsman's consciousness is trapped in the lord's authority. Yet like the water behind a dam, it breaks free to flow to its lowest point. Even without Hegel blatantly naming the low point, obviously, it is the body.

Hegel penned the next stage of this dynamic, detecting in it the start of a reversal. He wrote that the "bondsman . . . through his service rids himself of attachment to natural existence by working on it" (117). So with every act of labor and each object created, the bondsman "becomes conscious of what he truly is" and "comes to see in the independent being [of the object] its own independence" (119). In other words, the bondsman realizes they can create objects, to hew stone, hammer metal, tie rope and channel steam, in essence to create things that inadvertently forces a realization. *I stand above and apart from nature.* They know now they can destroy and re-create matter in its own image. Armed with evidence of their strength, they attack the former lord, who has been weakened by dependency. A new fight ensues. The bondsman triumphs and is the new lord. The roles are reversed. History spins like a roulette wheel.

Taking Cross's "Negro-to-Black Conversion Experience," the position in the body for both Hegel and Cross *is the return address*, the body is where alienation begins. After the lord and bondsman reverse places, the body is where alienation ends but in renewed consciousness. The five senses pour into a reflecting pool. You can see yourself again.

Hegel follows the bondsman's alienation, their entrapment in the lord and subsequent freedom through labor *back to their body*. Cross shows a Moral Shock, an Encounter, jolting Black consciousness to *flow to its body*. They balance on the same essential theme. And that one does not Return to the Body the same as when you left, but enlarged by social death, empowered by passing through the negative realm of alienation and agonizingly piecing together what reality is and is not. The new self is larger, it swallowed the whole night, inhaled distant stars, and gave birth to a sensitivity to the flow of time at one's fingertips.

The Return to the Body branches from Hegel and Cross to illuminate more books from within. The worker shines like a symbol on the treasure map, backlit by a candle. The body is the axle of history; empires and economies rise and fall as they spin upon it.

I grab *Marx-Engels Reader*, Marx famously took Hegel and "put him right side up," transforming his abstract vision into historical materialism. Imagine getting in that time machine and whooshing through a blur of twisted neon light and arriving in nineteenth-century Germany, as a young Marx strutted the street like John Travolta in *Staying Alive*. From what I read; the man was an arrogant genius. Yet he felt an incredible empathy for the poor. His large eyes darkened when obsessed by an idea. Friends would see his wild toss of hair, moving between books at the library.

Marx was the eldest son of Jewish family in Prussia that converted to Christianity, and in the 1830s went to college in Berlin. My man had no chill. He drank with friends at the Trier Tavern Club, fought in the streets, came home laughing with bloody teeth. The hellion was in as much upheaval as the world around him.

Marx read Hegel's "Lordship and Bondage" but projected the abstract philosophy into the real-life history played out between aristocrats and peasants, industrialists and workers. In the *Economic Manuscripts of 1844*, he wrote, "The alienation of the worker in his product means not only that his labour becomes an object, an external existence outside of him, independently as something alien to him, and that it becomes a power of its own confronting him" (72). You can hear in his prose Hegel's bondsman, who, after he loses to the lord "sets aside its own being-for-self" but "through work, becomes conscious of what he truly is" (118). The worker's work frees them. They become aware that they created the very world the capitalist owns. And they take it back. They overcome the ruling class superego.

The current, this flow of consciousness back to the body, is the force driving revolutions. In the 1848 "Manifesto of the Communist Party," Marx aimed for a larger audience. He crystallized this image of class conflict that turned the wheels of history:

> The history of all hitherto existing society is the history of class struggles. Freeman and slave, patrician and plebian, lord and serf, guild-master and journeyman, in a word, oppressor and oppressed, stood in constant opposition to one another, carried on an uninter-rupted, now hidden, now open fight, a fight that each time ended either in a revolutionary re-constitution of society at large, or in the common ruin of contending classes. (474)

Whether the Egyptian Empire or the Palaces of Versailles, the slave cabins of the American South, Starbucks cafés, and Amazon warehouses, workers unionize. Workers become aware that they are the true "lords." As long as a hierarchical society exploits its own, it alienates those who create everything we use and wear, drive, and eat; pressure builds to overcome the separation between consciousness and the body.

ꝣ ꝣ ꝣ

Buzzing, I took a joint and went to the roof. Today of all days was the time to see where a civilization that spirals so far from the body leads to. Fires in Canada engulfed whole forests and its smoke flowed 1,600 miles through the sky to paint New York orange.

Opening the roof door, I stepped outside and experienced the briny aftertaste. A tangerine haze submerged the city. *Piss Christ,* I thought. *It's like that photo of a crucifix in urine by Andres Serrano. Piss New York.*

I lit the joint, inhaled deeply, and blew. I surveyed Manhattan, the Mount Vesuvius of capitalism. Here money in motion finds its most gouache expression. New York City has more than eight million people, which means more than eight million stories. One story we are now wrestling with is the story of Global Warming. Industry dumps carbon in the sky, plastic in the ocean, and now plastic is in our blood. We are slowly drowning in the shit and piss of capitalism. Today is a special day because we can taste it in the Canadian wildfire smoke. It burns the eyes. Today is just the beginning. It is going to get worse.

The THC hit. My brain bobbed like a cork in water. Standing on the roof, I scanned New York's skyline from Brooklyn's One Hanson Place with the old-time clock to Manhattan's Freedom Tower that looked like a giant cut diamond. Next, I studied the Empire State Building, whose sharp point made it a hypodermic needle, and then Midtown's One Vanderbilt skyscraper that looked like huge glass plates fused into one. Each morning, we flowed from subways and buses, flowed down avenues, gushed into offices and construction sites, labs, and schools. We filled these buildings. We worked and our labor sent money up, up, up to regional managers, CEOs, investors, the 1 Percent. Rising like a giant tsunami of dollars, yen, yuan, pounds that filled the bank accounts of the wealthy.

I took another hit, and my head was an antenna catching strange visions. On my phone was geographer David Harvey's talk on Marxism but visualized as the Earth's water cycle. His sonorous British accent made me feel like a pupil at *Harry Potter's* Hogwarts school. Harvey said:

I've had the idea for some time to make Marx's ideas easy to follow. I tried to come up with a visualization . . . H_2O goes through a whole series of forms, starting as liquid in the ocean, condensation becomes vapor in the atmosphere, it is transported very fast through the atmosphere all over the place, it then starts to condense and form clouds and eventually forms precipitation, all sorts of forms of precipitation that can occur, snow, ice, rain, this precipitation falls on lands and takes various paths towards to oceans, some of the paths are very fast, some go very slowly, some hardly go at all, some of it gets locked up in ice caps . . . these transformations of form are what Marx calls metamorphosis. The definition of capital is value in motion. And exactly the same way that H_2O is in motion in this water-cycle, so capital is in perpetual motion.

I paused it and, flying high on the marijuana, I saw money, immense amounts of money, rising from the city into the sky like atmospheric rivers. Millions there. Billions in Midtown. Planetary wealth hovered over our heads in the bank accounts of the elite like heavy rain clouds; some of it "trickled down" in wages, tiny rivulets pooling into our pockets or direct deposit. We used it to pay rent, mortgage, and car notes. It was never enough.

I took another hit and looked up. I could see the 1 Percent dive from cloud to cloud like Walt Disney's Scrooge McDuck, who swims in gold coins and spits money like water. Here was Marx's core insight. Capital is money in motion. The wealthy poured their wealth into making more wealth. They bought more land, built more factories, more sweatshops, and mines. They made new businesses that needed cheap workers to trade labor for low wages. Capital's power to last across centuries was this ever-increasing expansion. It was like a hurricane that ripped lives from their moorings. It was like a flood that swept people into chaos.

I saw my decades in New York in a fast montage. Waves of gentrification lifted rents, lifted prices at the bodega, built condos my neighbors could not afford, new wine stores and cafés with expensive coffee and whites moving in from the Midwest. Each new wave made my neighbors struggle not to drown. Numbers rose above their thrashing hands.

I survived. I was like Basquiat. A scene from the 1996 film *Basquiat* flashed in my mind, where he crouched at a wall and sprayed "With The Big Money Crushed Into These Feet." He then looked at the building and imagined a man angling a surfboard on a wave. Later he met Benny Dalmau, a Nuyorican friend, and asked how long it took to get famous. Artists like me rode the wave of money, unleashed by the 1 Percent to make more money. Did Basquiat see the waves that David Harvey saw? Did he know what I know?

I stubbed the joint and threw it. I was so high my heart felt like a radio that received powerful signals that zapped the ventricles. I palmed my face and felt this life plus the lives that could have been. I embraced all of New York. I transformed into a single mom who dreaded the first of the month because she could not pay rent. I was a teen who sold sex for food. I mutated into a lonely, rich man who snorted coke in a dive bar bathroom. I was a seedy salesman who sold dinosaur bones to a wealthy patron who wanted to own deep time. I metamorphosed into a teen belt-tucking a gun because a crew chased me for money. I turned into an undocumented Mexican going from job to job, too tired to remember to eat. Eight million stories were for a second all mine.

All of it. The Totality.

How did capitalism trap us? I asked the marijuana spiking my blood to show me. Please, let me see it again.

Look at yourself.

I rubbed my gold ring. I pulled the label on my Banana Republic shirt. It read, "Made in Vietnam." I looked at my Macy's black shoes. I remembered that in my closet a dozen different "mes" of me were on the racks. Nuyorican Hipster Me. Professor Me. Sexy Date Me. Business Me. Hood Me. Burning Man Me. Sports Me.

Capitalism trapped us with the ability to buy new "mes" off the shelves. I stepped to the roof edge and surveyed Midtown where the mall at Columbus Circle would be and thought of the store windows that reflected passersby. Wherever I walked, multiple versions of me co-existed, each going in a different direction. You could walk many streets in New York lined with stores offering a new you.

See? See the Totality?

I did. I did. We worked to buy ourselves. The new self was a character in a larger story that moved toward the American Dream. We did not see that around us, the factories that made this dream, the oil we burned to drive to it and fly to it alongside the endless electricity to light and heat it was destroying the Earth. Only on days like today where we wore masks to protect our lungs from a faraway wildfire did we ask if the dream costs too much.

Look at your phone.

I had turned it off. The dark screen reflected my face like a dark puddle. Ah, here it was. Capitalism trapped us with our own reflection. We bought these tiny little screens, and they made us into millions of copycat Narcissus, who in the ancient Greek myth was trapped by his own reflection in a shallow pool. We also stared endlessly at ourselves. Our own social media. Our own algorithms.

We are drowning in ourselves.

I stepped back, put the phone away and thanked the marijuana for cleansing my vision. It is a mild psychedelic, but it let me feel the hidden forces around me. Terrifying at first. Going through the terror, I got to the other side more solid. It was the job of poets and activists to see beyond sight. I remembered Arthur Rimbaud's 1871 letter:

> The poet makes himself a seer by a long, prodigious, and rational disordering of all the senses. Every form of love, of suffering, of madness; he searches himself, he consumes all the poisons in him, and keeps only their quintessence. This is an unspeakable torture during which he needs all his faith and superhuman strength, and

during which he becomes the great patient, the great criminal, the great accursed—and the great learned one!—among men.—For he arrives at the unknown!"

Psychedelics transcended therapy. Consciousness is a gift, an ephemeral crack of light between the infinite dark before birth and the endless one after death. I had to aim this brief light at the world. And that was tradition. The more I taught and researched, the more authors I came across who struggled to stay clear. In literary criticism, a major conflict was how to measure the value of art. What is its place in the canon? How do we grade the relevance of an artist? How do we know whose consciousness is meaningful when so many traps exist for the mind? Fantasies can lead to delusion. Romanticism can justify prejudice. Nightmares paralyze imagination. Ideology can be an armor to protect a frail personality.

Psychedelics force the same questions. Beyond therapy, they lead us to touch the contours of hidden forces. Strangely, using psychedelics to peer through the ego to the vast surging energies was a classic gesture in Western Marxism. The tactic was expressed by György Lukács in his 1938 essay "Realism in the Balance," where he criticized the modernist fetish for fractured consciousness. Pushing back against self-dissolution, he urged, "If literature is a particular form by means of which objective reality is reflected, then it becomes of crucial importance for it to grasp reality as it truly is and not merely confining itself to reproducing whatever manifests itself immediately and, on the surface."

See it for what it truly is.

I took a last look at the orange sky over New York and breathed down, down, down into my lungs all the ash. I breathed Global Warming.

The marijuana receded from my blood. The once dizzy buzz faded to a background hum. I went back downstairs, cradling new ideas like a baby. New York has eight million stories. Now it has one more.

꙳ ꙳ ꙳

In my apartment, books were sprawled all over the floor. I put Marx back on the shelf. More questions came like a train rushing out of a station. So if a there's a "Negro-to-Black Conversion Experience" and a "Worker-to-Proletariat Conversion Experience," is there a "Woman-to-Feminist" one? Is there a "Closeted-to-Gay" one?

I remember women unspooling stories across my life. Like when Mom drove on a highway in sheets of rain, following red brake lights in front, retelling stories of coming of age in New York. How she shaped herself to fit what men wanted. It was a game whose rewards hid the costs. Say, when a friend in a numb metronome tone recounted a rape. Say, when I interviewed a genocide refugee and her eyes welled up with tears as she pointed to the desert where she had been ripped apart by a gang of men.

Patriarchy is deadly. Violence glues it to our lives. I hear it in hushed confessions. I see it in news reports of sexual trafficking. I read it in the great authors that line the bookshelf. The image that rises from them is a vast edifice, a massive social pyramid of power in which men lift men, pass property and status through their last names, and grant freedoms to each other and justify it through misogynist ideology.

When did it start? Is it in our DNA? Is it from private property, the rise of agriculture? Sifting the ancient past is tricky business. What is obvious is that patriarchy splits women into sharp contrast: "good women" who obey male supremacy and are duly "rewarded" and "bad women"—those who don't and are punished. We see that division repeated but with new names; here it's the saintly Madonna versus the whore, the Fallen Woman versus the Damsel in Distress, Tip Drill versus Wifey, the Puta Coño to the Hermana, the dyke or transwoman versus the "real woman."

Women always rebel. Most are lost in time. Taking the world history book from the shelf, you can flip through and literally see images of women toiling in obscurity, their lives like braille on the page. You can touch with a fingertip a sentence that pulses with their breath. You can feel them chafe against patriarchy. Maybe they met in secret and danced naked.

Maybe they shared herbs to induce abortions. Or ointments to heal after birth. When war, famine, or chaos shook their worlds, they were scapegoated as witches and burned alive as if the screams would be swallowed by other women to replace their voices.

Peeling their stories, a warm core reappears. The body again. The Return to the Body seems now like a crisscrossing interwoven stream, touching the spines of these books, lighting each one with liquidated sun.

Much of modern Feminist writing encircles the body, driving a return to it. One of the strong and long-standing themes is the struggle to untangle oneself from false images. Picking up Mary Wollstonecraft's 1792 *A Vindication of the Rights of Women*, one reads, "Taught from their infancy that beauty is woman's scepter, the mind shapes itself to the body, and, roaming round its gilt cage, only seeks to adorn its prison" (46). Again, the metaphor of imprisonment in a controlling image. One hundred and fifty years later, philosopher Simone De Beauvoir repeated that in her classic 1942 book, *The Second Sex*:

> The myth of woman . . . is a static myth . . . Thus against the dispersed, contingent, and multiple existences of actual women, mythical thought opposes the Eternal Feminine, unique and changeless. If the definition provided for this concept is contradicted by the behavior of flesh-and-blood women, it is the latter who are wrong: we are told not that Femininity is a false entity but that the women concerned are not feminine. (1407)

Again, we see the conflict. Inside that static phantom of the Eternal Feminine is the messy, complex, and fluid reality of living people.

A sort of psychological amputation occurs when the desires one has are illegal and out of fear of punishment, one saws off truths until a puppet is left dangling on strings held by men.

Oddly enough, it was Christopher Hitchens, a longtime Leftist, who in 1984 appeared on the arch-Conservative William Buckley's show *Firing Line*. He summed up in a pithy way how the Return to the Body in the early suffragette movement embraced the flesh in such a passionate way that it scared English society.

He debated Conservative writer Emmett Tyrrell Jr. of *The American Spectator*. Hitchens looked coyly at Buckley and Tyrrell, then opined on a favorite book, *The Strange Death of Liberal England*: "It's a wonderful evocation of pre-First World War Britain, when the old system, which was a liberal one, came under tremendous shocks"—he pinched his forefinger and thumb as if to catch a thought—"from the movement of women's suffrage, the movement to disengage from Ireland, and the rise of organized labor." His eyes glazed briefly as if seeing old England. "And in the chapter on women's suffrage, he described beautifully all the morbid symptoms that appear when a long repressed, especially sexually repressed group begins to take their own measure." He shot a glance at Tyrell. "The suffragette movement . . . was attacked by all kinds of people for its weirdness, the way women started to dress as men, neglect their families, behave promiscuously, and many of these symptoms"—he shook his eyes as if in awe—"up to and including suicide, were indeed present, but when the air cleared one could see that was the result of the original repression." The two Conservatives sat back and struggled to respond.

What is important is that his vignette of Britain shows how the repressed returns in a feverish rage. The parts, censored, the truths cut are recovered and embraced to the point of revolutionary fetishism. Desire beyond patriarchal monogamy becomes "Free Love." Glimpses of nonbinary sexuality in dress. Going on "strike" against the drudgery of domestic labor.

Looking at women writers in the United States, class and sex are tied to racism. Again, authors circled the body. In the 1975 choreopoem, *For Colored Girls Who Have Considered Suicide When the Rainbow Is Enuf*, Ntozake Shange wrote as the Lady in Orange, "ever since i realized there waz someone callt a colored girl an evil woman a bitch or a nag i been tryin not to be that & leave bitterness in somebody else's cup" (56). Twenty-five years later, Patricia Hill Collins published in 2000 *Black Feminist Thought*, which cataloged sexist imagery. She wrote, "Portraying African-American women as stereotypical mammies, matriarchs, welfare recipients, and hot mommas helps justify U.S. Black women's oppression. Challenging these controlling images has long been a core theme in Black Feminist thought" (76). What comes when the body shatters the "controlling images" is a rapid, volcanic identity change.

Black Panther leader Kathleen Cleaver said the same to a reporter. She pointed to friends sporting afros. "All of us were born with our hair like this"—she creased her forehead looking for words—"because it's natural. The reason for it you might say is there's a new awareness among Black people that their own natural physical appearance is beautiful." The video cut to handsome brothas and jaw-dropping sistahs. "For years we were taught that only white is beautiful. Only straight hair, light eyes, light skin was beautiful, and so Black women would try everything to straighten their hair and lighten their skin to look like white women." She steepled her hands and leaned into the camera. "This has changed because Black people are aware and white people are too. Now white people want natural wigs like this." She pointed to her own reddish afro. "Dig it? Isn't it beautiful?" She smiled as her sisters let out a bright, fluttering laugh.

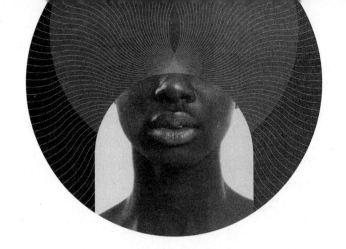

THE BODY ELECTRIC

SO, IT'S TRUE. THE BODY is the axle of history. Too many of us have pressed words to flesh and felt its flow. Hegel knew. Cross knows. De Beauvoir knew. Shange knew. Unnamed slaves knew and wrote testimony in fire.

It seems the cost of civilization is life in a pyramid of mirrors, where the powerful are reflected all around us until we see them inside too. Transference shatters this pyramid. It is an earthquake in muscle and nerve, mind and memory. When glistening shards fall to our feet, our vision is freed from mirrors and comes home to the body.

I know this from the protests I marched in. Let it be Occupy or Me Too, BLM, or Fuck Trump, the river of people waving signs and singing and chanting on long Manhattan avenues. We shouted the name of our real pain, our real hope. Above were corporate signs for McDonald's, Macy's, Bank of America, CNN, Walgreens, Walmart, Tiffany. Each one was like a magnet trying to levitate us back into the American Dream. We waved our own signs, sang, and marched, and fought to live in our bodies.

If what I see before me is right, if the Return to the Body is a salient concept, then the millions of us were ultimately testifying on behalf of it. Our exiled consciousness was like in Cross, like in Hegel, forcing its way past the ruling class superego, back home. We are not the first and certainly not the last.

Yet the sense that life is elsewhere is an uneasiness that poets have written about for centuries. In Rainer Maria Rilke's 1910 *The Notebooks of Malte Laurids Brigge*, a poetic, surreal novella, he penned a passage that captured this malaise:

> Is it possible that the entire history of the world has been misunderstood? Is it possible that we have the past all wrong, because we have always spoken of the masses, exactly as if we were describing a great throng of people, rather than speaking of the one man they were all gathered around—because he was a stranger and was dying?" (16)

What if the stranger who was dying was us? What if ideology is a veil of shadows? And breath, a midnight breeze? What if under all we think and speak is the heart, pulsing a message in Morse code?

The final book I pull from the shelf is Walt Whitman's *Song of Myself*. I love this poem so much. I even sniff its pages. Many authors on my shelves I adore and am deeply loyal to, but none say the essential truth like Whitman. Not Octavio Paz. Not Toni Morrison. Not André Breton. Not Homer.

Whitman unbuttoned his shirt and bared his juicy, giant heart like an ear to the universe. The truth he heard was, "I contain multitudes." If he were alive today, how would he say it? What would it sound like? I think it would be this:

> The body says, I am born and I die. I am male and female. I am trans. I am a gust of atoms blowing through the void. I love and I hate. I kill and I give birth. I am the past. I'm here with you now. I am lost in the horizon. I am a song blown from the mouth. I am shit and semen and placenta. I am many colors: brown and toffee, obsidian and pale. I am

short and tall, strong and sick. I am electricity in a moist brain. I am the memory my children hold and laugh with and cry over and cherish. I am the memory of my parents, forgiving and asking forgiveness. I am straight and gay and I am the unnamable flow of love between. I am the body! The body! The body! I belong to no one. I am your slave. I am your lord. I am the infinite space between words kept in motion by the flow of blood. I am food and drink in my stomach. I am a fart and a cough. I am a first breath and the last. I am sky. I am the reflection on the pupil of my lover, falling in dark wells to the living light of the mind. I am a sculpture of touches pressed on the soft clay of flesh that in time becomes a monster or saint. I am confused. I hope. I wonder what meaning life has? I live the answer, without knowing it. I am me. I am us. I was here. I will be again. I am. I am. I am.

Here is the body. From it comes all and all can't contain it. Wherever I turn, I see it. Civilization chops, saran wraps, packages, and puts a price tag on the body. Gods are stuffed down its throat and eyes. Money is poured into its stomach.

What is left is a small thing, a shadow in a cave, a hologram on the surface of breath.

§ § §

I put all the books away. I stuff Cross's essay between other essays. Sighing, I say "thank you" to all my mentors, the living and the dead, who taught me today.

Knowing what I know. We have to Return to the Body. We have to be in communion. All the ancestors will be dancing with us, like a duet with a cloud, like grinding hips on a breeze, or kissing a thunderstorm. The heartbeat is the way home.

PART
THREE

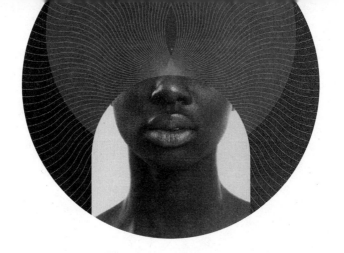

LUCY IN THE SKY
WITH DIAMONDS

DO I TAKE THIS TAB OF LSD, or not?

Inside the tiny paper square on my fingertip were chemicals strong enough to induce synesthesia. If I was lucky, a loss of self. Colors would melt. Sound would inflate me like a balloon. If I licked it, let it soak into brain tissue, buried versions of myself would be free to take shape in my mind. Like ghosts. Boo!

In a few hours, I was going to research drug history at the American Museum of Natural History. Oh, lysergic acid diethylamide. Do I or not? Half the fun of LSD was the challenge of tripping in odd places: a favorite park, a steamy porta-potty at Burning Man or the immersive art at Hall de Lumières. Chemical eyes perceive patterns within patterns spiraling in an infinite horizon that explains everything in one fell swoop.

But I had a job to do. Today I dive into psychedelic history to get clear answers to some questions: What role can they play today? How can they induce Collective Transference that revitalizes our breath, muscle, and brain? How can psychedelics go beyond one-on-one therapy and spin the roulette wheel of history, gamble with power, and win a future?

Ever since my first talk at Horizons, the annual psychedelics conference in New York, the Psychedelic Renaissance has grown like a late-night Brooklyn block party. Everyone's starting to show up, sneaking agendas in like flasks of whiskey in a coat pocket. Which is good and bad.

The media stampede to cover all things psychedelic means that for each sincere activist pushing legislation, there's a self-righteous gatekeeper yelling in Zoom meetings. For every Person of Color starting a ketamine clinic and doing outreach, there's one selling their color to white organizations who need a token. None of it is surprising.

Sometimes, I play back an interview I did, and creeping into my voice is the breathless panting of a zealot. It is like I saw Jesus at the club tossing MDMA pills at partygoers' mouths and turning bottles of water into wine. I became a true believer. I did not notice until it was too late that the Psychedelic Renaissance morphed into a Millenarian Cult. The rhetoric of radical change was more intoxicating than the drugs. It hit me that if someone built a statue of the LSD molecule, tens of thousands would bow down before it, praising it with hosannas.

The de facto leader of the Psychedelic Renaissance, Rick Doblin, founder of MAPS, also talked in millennial bombast. On the laptop, I saw his interview with *Psyche*. Leaning in a chair, he said, "We need a world of net-zero trauma. If we can globalize access to psychedelic healing, destigmatize it, and globalize this post-prohibition world, by 2050, a little bit less than another thirty-five years, we should have a net-zero trauma world. And also, we do need a shift from fundamentalism to mysticism. So we got people killing each other over

religious ideas and you know"—he motioned with his hands a plain-
tive gesture—"you can't force anybody to have these experiences, but
hopefully if we have enough of a cultural context where people have
had psychedelic mystical, unitive experiences that we will see a move
from fundamentalism, which is literalism to symbolic metaphorical
mysticism, so hopefully that's where will be at by 2050."

Pressing pause, I looked closer and closer at the LSD on my finger
as if a magnifying glass and could imagine, fifty-five years ago, my mom
studying an LSD tab in her hand, too, wondering if she was going to
make the jump. She did and often talked of psychedelic use in the
'60s. She, too, believed that some Great Spirit had descended upon
the world that would end war, poverty, and racism, in part because
visions inspired by psychedelics. They were of a love so powerful you
could see around you, hands, endless hands reaching for the same
truth. We all are one humanity.

I put the LSD down. It did not work then. Wars left a bloody
bomb-cratered trail from Vietnam to Iraq to Yemen to the Congo and
Ukraine. Poverty deepened. How can it work now? What happened?
What did not happen?

What I needed to know was how this moment was different. The
Medical Model in which MDMA and maybe later LSD and psilocybin
were legalized for therapy was openly talked about as a Trojan horse.
The hope was that wide-sweeping cultural change would be the real
"side effect." Once psychedelics are welcomed into the mainstream,
their "mind-manifesting power" would cause the downfall of fundamentalism. Which is why legalization was so vital. It was slow incremental work inside the system that would get to a net-zero trauma
civilization. It would not be like the 1960s. We would not make the
same mistakes.

I put my elbows on the table and studied the tab. So much hope,
so much money, so many lives balanced on these chemicals. Today's

Psychedelic Renaissance is the second time in American history that LSD and mushrooms alongside ayahuasca and peyote were popping up on the evening news or daytime television. Except in those conversations they were shorn of utopian politics. They were strictly medicines given by therapists to treat depression or addiction. They were cool. They were safe. Most importantly, America was safe from them.

In the late '60s, America was both terrified of LSD and prayed to LSD. It was like the opening of Charles Dickens's 1859 novel, *A Tale of Two Cities*, except it was *The Tale of Two Drugs* with completely opposite stories about LSD. If Dickens were alive, he'd write, "It opened the Doors of Perception. It caused madness. It unveiled Heaven on Earth. It transformed us into sinners. It could bring peace. It could unleash the Dogs of War. It was a step forward by science. It cast us back into caves."

What I do know is that for those I love, my mom, my friends, even the strangers I met over the years at festivals or in parks, LSD and psychedelics in general were a godsend. They may have not "saved" us, but they saved us from being brainwashed by the system. They gave us breathing space to figure out our lives.

What I know is that in 1967, the Summer of Love, LSD and magic mushrooms transported a generation back to their bodies. The Be-Ins, drums circles, the "Turn on, tune in, drop out," the laced sugar cubes, the Free Love and "Fuck War"; all of it was a once in a millennia confluence of historical forces that positioned psychedelics as a tool for liberation. The question was, Could it happen again?

I looked from the LSD to the bookshelves again, to see the Return to the Body seeping from the Black Literary Canon part of my library into the Counterculture section. Here *Storming Heaven* by Jay Stevens sat next to *Ransoming Pagan Babies* by Warren Hinckle near *Heads* by Jesse Jarnow, within each one glowed scenes of Collective Transference, where repressed truths surged like a wave. When the wave receded, a new person remained, cleansed of who they had been before, touching their face without a mask, without the chastity belt of religion and feeling their bodies like newborn babies.

I opened a '60s history book and saw colorful photos of youth dancing barefoot, Indian beads swinging, arms loose like rag dolls. Joy was a victory against overwhelming odds. Every Hippie, smiling as they tongued an LSD sugar cube, challenged the global superpower. They discovered in their minds was the American superego in all its glory, all its Stars and Stripes, its bald eagle and atomic bomb, its "No Coloreds" signs, its clean white skin and clean white homes and clean white teeth, its big cars and new TV set, its backyard grills, its pools, its dread of Communism, its God Bless America, all of it washed away like watercolors from a canvas by a tab of acid.

Sometimes, I take my elderly mentors from the '68 generation to a pub or get them high in the park. Many are dying nowadays. In their stories, LSD is like the sun's reflection on the sea. The truth blinded them. After the trip, the real world looked like a prop town in a Western movie. It was an empty front but inside was nothing.

I picked up the tab again. This damn little thing. And it was all an accident.

※ ※ ※

The LSD tab on my fingertip is a freak accident. I knew its origin by heart. On the screen was a photo of a man with an oblong face, arched eyebrows, and a focused look, posing in a lab coat. Swiss chemist Albert Hoffman mixed chemicals in the search for a respiratory stimulant. In 1938, he came across lysergic acid diethylamide but wasn't impressed and put it away. Five years later in 1943 he checked it again, accidentally smudged a bit on his fingers, and boom!

Hoffman said a "dreamlike" state overwhelmed him. Days later, April 19, Hoffman took LSD on purpose and bicycled home, woozy and loopy.

He wrote, "Kaleidoscopic, fantastic images surged in on me, alternating, variegated, opening and then closing themselves in circles and spirals, exploding in colored fountains, rearranging and hybridizing themselves in constant flux." His mind was a flower opening to a sunrise.

Sandoz Pharmaceuticals, who employed Hoffman, marketed LSD under the name Delysid. In the 1950s, therapists experimented with it as a treatment for mental health problems. In the '50s! *Ozzie and Harriet. Father Knows Best.* McCarthyism. Legal racial segregation. You know, the '50s!

It was easy because LSD, or Delysid, was a blank slate; it had no story, no ideological baggage. Alongside it was magic mushrooms, an old sacrament in Mexican villages, famously shared by medicine woman María Sabina. White researchers like Hoffman traveled to Mexico, sat in ceremony, and later synthesized it. Media caught on. More followed. Bill Wilson, co-founder of Alcoholics Anonymous, said it helped addicts "surrender" to healing. Hollywood actor Cary Grant dosed and said he was "reborn." *Time* ran cheering essays on the new miracle drugs; first was a 1954 article titled "Dream Stuff" saying it "can be of great benefit to mental patients," followed by a 1957 article called "Seeking the Magic Mushroom," and again in 1960, another piece titled "The Psyche in 3-D" about Hollywood celebs imbibing the wonder drug under a doctor's careful watch.

Doesn't all this sound familiar? Medical packaging? Check. Elites using it openly? Check. Mainstream media cheerleading? Check.

I so want to go back in time, tiptoe up on Hoffman, yank his face and discover it was a rubber mask worn by Doblin. I'll be like, "Rick, it was you the whole time!" He'd laugh, press a button on his coat, and teleport to another dimension.

Psychedelic therapy goes back to the '50s. Why was it so accepted then? I pull Michele Dillon's *Introduction to Sociological Theory* and flip to the section on Talcott Parsons. He was an American sociologist at Harvard who founded Structural Functionalism. Imagine a mechanic studying an engine turning wheels. Parsons peeked under the hood of everyday life to see what makes society run. First is *Adaptation* or how a culture adapts people to the environment. His example was farms—kids did not need schools to adapt to milking cows and shoveling shit. City families did need schools to adapt to an industrial economy that needed literate workers who could read blueprints and fix machines. Next is *Goal Attainment*, as in, what are the ideals we try to live—say, the American Dream of a new house, marriage, and heterosexuality. Third is *Integration*, where social norms are expressed and enforced by authorities, maybe a cop or priest or teacher. Finally, we have *Pattern Maintenance*, in which social values are transmitted to people via institutions that are both physical, like a school or church or sports games, and ceremonial, as in the Pledge of Allegiance or a wedding.

Using these four definitions, Parsons broke down the intricate, multilevel, moving pieces of society to the smallest atom that he called a *Unit Act*. The components of a Unit Act are first, social actors or someone doing something; second, a goal, some tangible effect; third, a physical place for the action to happen; and fourth, the positive social value that it upholds, re-creates, embodies.

Psychedelics was in the 1950s a Unit Act. Let's circle back to Set, Setting, and Container in which Set is the mental state of the tripper. Are they trying to heal trauma, get artistic spark, or feel vibes at a music event? Setting is the physical locale, a retreat in Costa Rica or underground rave or CIA torture chamber. Finally, the Container is the ideological frame that makes meaning of the psychedelic trip. In therapy the trip is for a healed self. If you are an Aztec king, the trip reinforces belief in his own divine rule. What it means is Set, Setting, and Container are a subset of the larger Unit Act; in other words, the trip takes place in and has meaning within a larger culture.

||||||||||||||||||||||||||||||||||||||||||||||||||||||||||||||||||||||||||||||||||||||||||||||||||||||||||||||||||

SET, SETTING, CONTAINER

Culture shapes a trip. In the book *American Trip: Set and Setting and the Psychedelic Experience in the Twentieth Century* author Ido Hartogsohn writes, "We should pay closer attention to how psychedelic experiences are shaped, not just at the individual level . . . but also more broadly at the collective level, based on the sociopolitical conditions of place and time" (8). Hartogsohn contrasts what he calls the American Trip with other cultures, mostly tribal, that use chemicals to heal or as part of a rite of passage. In each one, it functioned to maintain society.

LSD and mushrooms in the '50s were seen as a tool of Adaptation and Integration. They were a miracle cure to help the maladapted, like drunks, adapt and integrate into working life. They were first advertised as a way to keep the status quo. It was *functional*, much like getting a broken bone set or a blood infusion. And then LSD "escaped the lab."

||||||||||||||||||||||||||||||||||||||||||||||||||||||||||||||||||||||||||||||||||||||||||||||||||||||||||||||||||

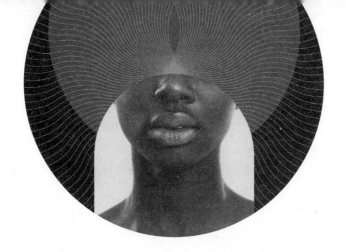

PUTTING FLOWERS IN GUN BARRELS

A ROW OF TABS ON my computer screen, and each one is a puzzle piece that fits together into a larger portrait of tragedy. LSD and mushrooms were transformed from a boutique medicine into a chemical demon that scourged America.

Psychedelics caught in the changing tides. Underneath the 1950s and early 1960s was a strong undercurrent. The youth chafed under the Silent Generation. They saw the US spill blood in Korea and Vietnam, deny Black people the right to vote or public accommodations, and the rank hypocrisy of the family. A pair of scientists stoked this discontent to white hot intensity. In 1960, Timothy Leary and Richard Alpert began the Harvard Psilocybin Project. Harvard of all places!

In the photos, Leary has a twinkle in his eye like a pool hall hustler. Alpert wears thick black glasses and a cherubic smile, already radiating a mesmerizing innocence. They ordered psilocybin from Sandoz Pharmaceuticals and gave it to hundreds of people, students, prisoners—hell, if they saw a passing space alien in a hubcap shaped–UFO, they'd throw it a tab. They. Gave. It. To. Everyone. They themselves did a biblical amount of LSD and psilocybin. They might as well have had brain surgery and told the doctor to firehose their skulls.

Leary and Alpert saw psychedelics as more than a tool to help the individual adapt and integrate into society. They believed it could cure the American mind, obsessed as it was with white supremacy and fighting Communism. The US was just fifteen years past World War II. The nation's power elite, a term coined by C. Wright Mills in his 1956 book, *The Power Elite*, was on high alert. Soldiers in uniform and businessmen in suits lumbered through the halls of Washington, DC, and vowed to defend the West against Communist Soviet Union. World War II may be over but war continued. War was forever.

What Leary and Alpert, among many others, saw was that humanity had entered a new epoch with the atomic bomb. We could now destroy ourselves. The enemy was no longer the enemy. Now, war itself was the enemy.

Beneath the headlines, Leary, and Alpert probably—I can't say this for certain, but it's a hunch—saw a lot of traumatized WWII veterans. Not in official practice. I mean in private life. I think they knew men who drank and beat their wives and kids because, in their minds, they never left the war. How many woke up screaming in a cold sweat because they couldn't stop seeing a friend blown to bits by a Nazi grenade?

This was the America that Leary and Alpert saw. It was sick with racism, militarism, and materialism and needed healing. They pushed LSD and psilocybin beyond the Medical Model. What they did was sloppy. In some cases, stupid and careless, but it was part of a larger social movement, a wave of discontent, a pressure building in the private lives of people that exploded in public.

In an interview, Alpert responded to critics. In a charming tone, he said, "All they could see were the problems and the fears of society but none of the potential, none of the positive questions about what is Man to do next and what possibility that LSD might hold." He moved his hand forward as if offering a gift. "They are not even interested in that. They are so committed to the fact that this society is the way it is and that's all you can expect." He looked down as if gathering strength. "I call that having a vested interest in the ongoing game, and if you are invested in the ongoing game, you'll be frightened by anything that might change it."

They took psychedelics with students. Two went to a mental hospital from their trips. Harvard turned on Leary and Alpert. Leary left, said he was done with the "science" and began a career as a psychedelic evangelical, proclaiming the good word of LSD. Alpert was fired and went on a spiritual journey to India, met a guru, turned inward, then outward, and renamed himself Ram Dass. His 1970 book, *Be Here Now,* was a Hippie holy text. They brought psychedelics to a rising wave of rebellious youth, seeking answers to the multiple crises rocking America—the Vietnam War, racism, the Sexual Revolution— saying in essence, here is how to free your mind, or as Leary branded it, "Turn on, tune in, drop out."

LSD and psilocybin did not "escape the lab"; Leary hurled it out with the force of an NFL quarterback. It soared across the firmament like a bright meteor that crash-landed in the run-down bohemian neighborhood of San Francisco's Haight-Ashbury. Jay Stevens recounts in *Storming Heaven,* his tour de force of LSD history, that by 1965, the paint-peeled homes and trashy streets of the Haight were a haven for Beats, then Hippies, who built an alternate America of weed, LSD, and Free Love. The Hippie grapevine went into overdrive, and ears picked up along wind-swept highways and art gatherings, beach parties and jails. Celestial Energy was hot at the Haight.

My secret pleasure is watching '60s newsreels of Haight-Ashbury bus tours. Older staid visitors in suits and dresses peered from windows at Hippies lounging on sidewalks. The bus driver said, "It is the belief of the people who live in the area that we of the middle class or the upper class have done a very poor job of running our government, running our way of life." Riders smiled nervously as they read pamphlets with street slang. On the sidewalk, couples in ponchos or Native beads waved. Or one time they held up mirrors so tourists saw reflections of themselves staring in disgust.

Returning to Parsons, when LSD was thrown from the lab to the streets, it was thrown out of the functional "story," out of the role it played as a medicine. It was no longer a Unit Act of the status quo. No helping drunks off the bottle. No ecstatic testimonials from Hollywood celebs or swooning *Time* essays. LSD no longer helped Americans adapt or integrate into the mainstream. Now authorities saw it as a threat. Psychiatrists, cops, and politicians looked on in horror as LSD grew horns and a tail and prodded poor American youth with a fiery pitchfork into debauchery, Communism, and race mixing.

Taking the 2009 textbook *Criminology* by Larry J. Siegel from the pile, I see in the first section how the history of psychedelics is a history of social control. The power elite, or in '60s parlance, the Establishment, had a consensus view of crime, in that "crimes are behaviors believed to be repugnant to all elements of society" (16). The belief is that crime causes social harm and "behaviors that are harmful to other people and society in general must be controlled" (16). The youth seemed to hurt themselves with LSD. Upstanding boys left the church, refused the draft, and peered through Eastern religions to look for guidance. Virginal girls left home, danced barefoot in the rain, took many lovers, and worse, mixed with other races.

Criminologists have long known that class conflict shapes how we perceive crime. Again Siegel gives a definition of the Marxist-inspired conflict view and sees "society as a collection of diverse groups—owners, workers, professional students—who are in constant and continuing conflict. Groups able to assert their political power use the law and the criminal justice system to advance their economic and social position" (17). He sums it up in a hard-hitting sentence: "Crime . . . is a political concept." So even though the chemical composition of LSD did not change at all, the role it played went into a complete reversal once it left the therapist office, the lab, the academy, and private Hollywood parties and hit the street.

If you stop at "The Man says LSD is bad," you will miss the beauty of what happened. Again using Parson's terminology, Hippies made LSD into a *Unit Act of the Counterculture*; it was functional. It helped newcomers to the Haight, who grew up "square," in *Father Knows Best*–type nuclear families, adapt to communal living and attain the goals of peace, art, and open love. Again, in *Storming Heaven*, Stevens vividly described it:

> At first the hippies used LSD as a deconditioning agent . . . That American society was manipulative was one the Haight's basic tenets. LSD put this into perspective . . . it opened up the possibility of reprogramming oneself; using LSD the games could be examined, the defenses leveled, and better strategies adopted. The word on Haight Street was that a few good acid trips were the equivalent of three years of analysis. (300)

LSD was "good." LSD was Sunday church or the Pledge of Allegiance or rather a Pledge to the Age of Aquarius. It was a functional act for the Counterculture. It gave the artists and youth a way to embody new ideals, values that were the exact opposite of the ones hammered into their brains since birth.

Why is this important? Remembering what Mom told me, what elderly mentors told me, and what I saw in history was that those driven to the Haight or what Hippie town they could find were deeply

wounded by America. They were curious about truth outside broad-
cast TV. They were branded with shame for sexual desire. Artists like
Allen Ginsberg were exiled for poetry that mixed the profane and
sacred. They were students, disgusted with American bombs blasting Vietnamese into chunks of meat. Or they were kids, beaten and
abused by parents, fleeing into the streets, recreating with strangers—
also sunburned, hungry, and hardened—a family that, however poor,
at least let them live in peace.

A powerful testimony of the orphans at the core of the Counterculture came from Joan Didion. She began her 1968 book of essays,
Slouching Towards Bethlehem, with the sentence, "The center was not
holding" and followed it with a crushing description of America, hol-
lowed out and helpless. Under billboards promising a new life, teens
passed jugs of wine, families ran from debt, homes were vacated in a
rush, adults changed their names. Some of these vagabonds, Didion
saw, made it to the Haight:

> We were seeing the desperate attempt of a handful of pathetically
> unequipped children to create a community in a social vacuum. Once
> we had seen these children, we could no longer overlook the vacuum,
> no longer pretend that the society's atomization could be reversed. (84)

Stevens added to this in *Storming Heaven* when he quoted social scientist Helen Swick Perry, calling the Haight a "delta of a river," a pooling
of the "unrooted sediment of America" that "washed ashore" (301). The
United States quietly disintegrated. Debris blew along the land.

Imagine on a highway, a young white man coming from nowhere,
going nowhere. He slept under an overpass, woke up and climbed the
hill. Cold dawn was a blessed numbness. Last night's LSD made the
sunrise look like an atomic bomb in slow motion. He asked Jesus to
let him melt like an atomic test dummy. He remembered what friends
told him. Go West. Everyone was going West. To Haight-Ashbury. The

name rang like a church bell. He slapped dust off his jeans and followed his long shadow, pointing like a compass needle to the Pacific Ocean.

When I put down the books, I feel for that generation great gratitude and reverence but also sadness. They ran from pain and tried to find salvation in each other. What they revealed was a truth that had been buried like a bone at a crime scene. What made LSD a danger was its role in Transference, in particular Collective Transference because it showed the United States was built on lies.

I took *The Language of Psycho-Analysis* from the shelf again to reread the entry on Transference, "Actualisation of unconscious wishes . . . infantile prototypes re-emerge and are experienced with a strong sensation of immediacy" (455). Again, I reread the lines, "Freud stresses that it is connected with 'prototypes' or imagos (chiefly the imago of the father, but also of the mother, brother, etc.): the doctor is inserted 'into one of the psychical "series" in which the patient has already formed,'" and further down, "Transference on to the person of the physician is triggered off precisely at the moment when particularly important repressed contents are in danger of being revealed" (458). I closed it again with a snap and had to ask, Who or what played the role of the "prototype" or "imago" that echoed a parent or family or authority? Who did the Hippies *transfer* their collective generational conflict on?

In the book pile, I found James Baldwin's essay, "No Name in the Street," where he visited Haight-Ashbury and saw who the Hippies used as a blank screen for Transference. It was the skeletons in America's unconscious. The Native American, Black, and Latino were the "parental figures" that guilt and the hope for salvation were transferred onto like a blank movie screen. Baldwin wrote:

I next came to San Francisco at the time of the flower children . . .
Their flowers had the validity, at least, of existing in direct challenge

to the romance of the gun; their gentleness . . . was nevertheless a direct repudiation of the American adoration of violence . . . An historical wheel had come full circle. The descendants of the cowboys, who had slaughtered the Indians, the issue of those adventurers who had enslaved the blacks, wished to lay down their swords and shields. (547)

In rejecting John Wayne and embracing Native Americans, in rejecting the Ku Klux Klan and embracing Black people, white Hippies bypassed the American superego and, through cultural appropriation, returned to their bodies. They hugged, wildly, passionately the parts of themselves that had been censored or amputated by parents and schools, churches and sitcoms.

The Return to the Body in the Hippie movement was a large-scale breakdown of white supremacy. Psychedelics had real political and cultural effects that far surpassed one-on-one therapy with a doctor. Hippie culture idealized the very racial minorities being stereotyped by the white power structure. Which is amazing considering they grew up with books, films, and radio filled with caricatures: the eye-rolling darkie, sneaky Asian, horny Latin man, the sultry Dragon Lady, or shifty Jew, vengeful Arab, and savage Indian.

In real life, public racism was the pillar of America with real lynchings and real signs saying "No Jews," "No Mexicans," and "No Coloreds." White supremacy was fueled by Racial Projection, a dynamic defined in *The Language of Psycho-Analysis* as an "operation whereby qualities, feelings, wishes or even 'objects,' which the subject refuses to recognize or rejects in himself, are expelled from the self and located in another person or thing" (349). The projection of animal sexuality, violence, and heathen witchery onto non-white people was an act of creating a modern white ego by dividing from the self-representations of bodily instincts and *projecting* them onto the others. It is specifically an act of forced nonrecognition.

The Black Literary Canon is rife with authors calling out Racial Projection. W. E. B. Du Bois's Double-Consciousness is one of the earliest. In his 1903 *The Souls of Black Folk*, he wrote, "It is a peculiar sensation, this double-consciousness, this sense of always looking at one's self through the eyes of others, of measuring one's soul by the tape of a world that looks on in amused contempt and pity" (619). Twenty-four years later in 1927, E. Franklin Frazier added to Du Bois's Double-Consciousness with his essay "The Pathology of Race Prejudice," where he described the Southern white's Negro-Complex in which "the extremely repugnant system of dissociated ideas is projected upon some real or imaginary individual" (859). His analysis was added to in Nobel Prize winner Toni Morrison's classic 1987 novel, *Beloved*, where she writes on racists:

> White people believed that whatever the manners, under every dark skin was a jungle . . . red gums ready for their sweet white blood. In a way, he thought, they were right. The more colored people spent their strength trying to convince them how gentle they were, how clever and loving, how human, the more they used themselves up to persuade whites of something Negroes believed could not be questioned, the deeper and more tangled the jungle grew inside . . . It was the jungle white folks planted in them. And it grew. It spread. In, through and after life, it spread, until it invaded the whites who had made it. Touched them everyone. Changed and altered them. Made them bloody, silly, worse than even they wanted to be, so scared were they of the jungle they had made. The screaming baboon lived under their own white skin; the red gums were their own. (89)

Morrison reverses primitivist imagery, hollows out the content of "jungle" in white supremacist ideology as a metonymy of racial inferiority. She refills it like an empty Tupperware with its real content, which is violence, specifically the violence that follows projection.

In contrast to projection is Transference. Hippies reversed the dynamic by idealizing oppressed races, and the first step was reimagining them as family members. One way or another each became a "parental figure," so Native Americans were "elders of the land," South Asian Indians were "grandparents bearing ancient wisdom," and Black folks transformed into "brothers and sisters." Idealized family prototypes allowed for a Transference or the "actualisation of unconscious wishes" so that however obscured by racial romanticism, it led to a reembracing of the censored body, which had profound political consequences. The United States was a highly Christian, white supremacist, and heterosexual nation driven by capitalism and glued together by a middle-class ideal of monogamy, marriage, and a house mortgage. In short, it was under the spell of the American Dream. When eye-patch-wearing, beefy-armed journalist Warren Hinckle strode through the Haight, unlike other reporters, he did not dismiss the Hippies as dreamy idiots. In his 1967 essay "The Social History of the Hippies," he wrote clearly and candidly about the values undergirding the scene:

> The utopian sentiments of these hippies were not to be put down lightly. Hippies have a clear vision of a psychedelic community . . . [it] embodies a radical political philosophy: communal life, drastic restriction of private property, rejection of violence, creativity before consumption, freedom before authority . . . they take LSD and marijuana . . . enjoy sleeping nine to a room and three to a bed, seem to have free sex and guiltless minds, and can raise healthy children in dirty clothes. (154)

Putting his essay next to Baldwin's, the radicalism of that moment shines more powerfully. In small living room gatherings where LSD was dropped on tongues or in the large gatherings of Trip Journeys or the Be-Ins, a Collective Transference created a generation going in the opposite direction of the rest of the United States. It grew in force and

power, threatening to levitate the Pentagon by chanting om. Or stop
the Vietnam War by making young men put flowers in the gun barrels
of soldiers.

The rare incandescent joy of the '60s inspired some fine American writing. In his 1971 classic road trip memoir, *Fear and Loathing in
Las Vegas*, gonzo author Hunter S. Thompson etched a wild, wind-in-
your-hair portrait of the time. It is the classic "wave" section where he
reminisces:

> San Francisco in the middle sixties was a very special time and place
> to be a part of. Maybe it meant something. Maybe not, in the long
> run . . . but no explanation, no mix of words or music or memories
> can touch that sense of knowing that you were there and alive in that
> corner of time and the world . . . .

> I left the Fillmore half-crazy and, instead of going home, aimed the
> big 650 Lightning across the Bay Bridge at a hundred miles an hour . . .
> booming through the Treasure Island tunnel at the lights of Oakland
> and Berkeley and Richmond, not quite sure which turn-off to take
> when I got to the other end . . . but being absolutely certain that no
> matter which way I went I would come to a place where people were
> just as high and wild as I was: No doubt at all about that . . . .

> There was madness in any direction, at any hour. If not across
> the Bay, then up the Golden Gate or down 101 to Los Altos or La
> Honda . . . . You could strike sparks anywhere. There was a fantastic
> universal sense that whatever we were doing was right, that we were
> winning . . . .

> And that, I think, was the handle—that sense of inevitable victory
> over the forces of Old and Evil. Not in any mean or military sense,
> we didn't need that. Our energy would simply prevail. There was no
> point in fighting—on our side or theirs. We had all the momentum;
> we were riding the crest of a high and beautiful wave . . . . (127)

The Establishment freaked out. Bongo-drumming, free-sex-having, blissed-out "barbarians at the gate" were loving the world to peace. The '60s was a time of barbarians. Roaring on highways, the Hell's Angels, an outlaw biker gang, gave Middle America the middle finger. They beat up local townies, threw beer-and-acid-fueled parties with Ken Kesey, and gang raped. All this was chronicled by Thompson in his 1967 book, *Hell's Angels*. Classic barbarian stuff. Black Power replaced the Civil Rights Movement's Christian songs and American flags with afros, clenched fists, and guns. Yummy. Black barbarians. But Hippies struck two primal fears in Middle America. The first was patricide. White kids were transformed by psychedelics into monsters hell-bent on destroying the nation for some illusionary Age of Aquarius. The second was a kind of infanticide as even children were being sacrificed on the altar of LSD.

One terrifying scene came from Didion's already-mentioned essay "Slouching Towards Bethlehem." I can almost imagine her licking her thumb in glee as she stumbled on a Hippie family who cheerfully fed their five-year-old daughter LSD. Didion reported:

> When I finally find Otto he says, "I got something at my place that'll blow your mind," and when we get there, I see a child on the living-room floor, wearing a reefer coat, reading a comic book. She keeps licking her lips in concentration and the only off thing about her is that she's wearing white lipstick.
>
> "Five years old," Otto says. "On acid." (127)

And that's why LSD was a scapegoat. It made Hippies into victims of their own idealism. They needed to be rescued before they brought all of Western civilization crashing down into a pile of rubble. The criminalization of psychedelics let the Establishment off the hook. It could deny that the white youth who protested the Vietnam War or racial segregation or sexual hypocrisy or who dropped out of capitalism had legit reasons. No. It must be the LSD. The LSD made them mad. It's the LSD!

States led the charge, followed by the Feds, to push a Prohibition era for psychedelics. In 1966 *The Desert Sun* announced that California and Nevada criminalized LSD, with fines at $1,000 and a possible year in jail. Four years later, in 1970, Congress passed the Controlled Substances Act, which outlawed LSD absolutely.

Psychedelics lived on. A year after California banned it, Hippies gathered at the Human Be-In at Golden Gate Park. Nearly 30,000 listened to Timothy Leary and Allen Ginsberg exhort the new world glimpsed in kaleidoscope visions. The Be-In flowed into the 1968 Summer of Love. Dosed sugar cubes or tabs were placed on tongues across America like sacraments at New Age Holy Communion. Eyes spiraled like starry galaxies. Elevated from attachments to symbols and ego, trippers touched billowy clouds of Heaven.

Inevitably, the Establishment won. If you close your eyes, you'll hear "The Imperial March" from *Star Wars: The Empire Strikes Back*. Threatening horns. Evil bombast. Darth Vader takes off his mask, and it's President Nixon saying, "Public enemy number one is drug abuse." The vast pyramid of power that is the US government; from the apex of the White House, the Senate, the House to the state capitals to the small towns, it moved to crush the Psychedelic Movement. Medical research went underground. Acid heads, jailed.

"When it tipped over in America," said an elderly Albert Hoffman. "The miracle drug became a Satan drug." In the interview, he sighed heavily. "And this whole wonderful, beautiful development was interrupted because of the American story." It was a scene toward the end of *How to Change Your Mind* on Netflix. The host, a wizened Michael Pollan said that psychedelics went into the Dark Ages. Decades went by before a crack in the laws let a ray of hope in.

☙ ☙ ☙

"Happy Birthday to you," the crowd sang to Hoffman. He palmed his chest and waved at adoring fans in the hall. It was 2006. It was his 100th birthday. The gathering was a psychedelic research conference in Oslo, Sweden. At the end, they sent an open letter to governments all over to restart LSD research. The scene was from *How to Change Your Mind*. Next you see Dr. Peter Gasser, giddy at getting LSD from the Swedish Health Ministry and walking the streets, holding the first legal dose in decades.

I paused the video and leaned back. The scene had switched to Hoffman, who leaned on a cane. He visited Gasser after the Swedish state gave the greenlight for LSD research to give his blessing. Two years later, in 2008, Hoffman died.

The father of LSD teasingly called it his "problem child." He did not see the Psychedelic Renaissance. He died just as Drug War propaganda was thawing. I'll go out on a limb and say, he never saw the knee-slapping magic mushroom scene in 2007's *Knocked Up* when Seth Rogen ate caps and stems and had a shit-in-his-pants, full-blown panic attack at a Vegas circus show. Nor did Hoffman live to see *How to Change Your Mind*, where patients cried in relief with therapists. He missed officials in Oakland and Denver decriminalizing psychedelics. He visited Harvard to learn about new investment in psychedelic research.

If he had lived fifteen more years, he could have flown to Denver in 2023 to be honored at the psychedelic conference. Wheeled on stage, Hoffman would have been hugged by Doblin and loved by a stadium filled with nearly 13,000 adoring activists and researchers. He would have gotten his flowers.

I'm glad he didn't. I can imagine the wild, thundering applause as thousands hung on his every word like from an oracle. He would have doubled down on his reformist ideology, which would have driven the Psychedelic Movement further in the wrong direction. However much Hoffman saw on LSD, he was more blinded by hope.

My face reflected on the screen, and I held the LSD tab again. What a strange, horrific time it was born into. When Hoffman first tasted LSD and bicycled home on April 19, 1943, roughly eight hundred miles away in Poland, a handful of Jewish insurgents in the Warsaw Ghetto fought Nazis. It was a modern Siege of Masada. Each Jew who battled Nazis knew they would die. The odds were overwhelming. Face-to-face with death, they saw more clearly than Hoffman on LSD or his acolytes in the '60s Underground or today's Psychedelic Renaissance. The Jewish resistance against the Final Solution saw past hope. They did not fight to save their lives. They fought to save their dignity.

I hold this contradiction to my chest like an ice pack. Every year, psychedelic activists celebrate Bicycle Day on April 19, when Hoffman took his first LSD trip. It is a fun day filled with celebrations and events. Yet I think of World War II roaring like a tornado of steel around the euphoric bubble of LSD's birth. While Hoffman laid on his couch in the thrall of visions, not far away in France, soldiers ran into a rain of bullets. In London and Dresden, civilians ducked as air sirens wailed and search lights crisscrossed the skies to see a dark flock of bombers. After battles men hosed blood off tanks.

Can LSD stop war? The question takes on added weight because the discovery of LSD came in the bright light of the atomic bomb. As Hoffman pondered the meaning of LSD, more than 5,000 miles across the Atlantic Ocean in a dust-swept Los Alamos, New Mexico, Robert Oppenheimer led an army of construction workers and scientists to create the bomb before the Nazis.

In that brief window of time, humanity gained tools of titanic power, LSD and the atomic bomb. One exposed the infinite light of the mind and the latter put the explosive light of the sun at our fingertips. Hoffman realized LSD expanded consciousness and gave us a blessed glimpse of our human unity, the interconnectedness of life. Maybe it could save us from ourselves? At the same time, the bomb cast a giant mushroom shadow over the Earth. Today, tens of thousands of nuclear missiles sleep in silos, each one bearing a radioactive seed of apocalypse. Just one war could escalate into species suicide. Yet in this LSD tab on my fingertip were chemicals that let us transcend bloodlust. Which one would win out?

I do not trust Hoffman's legacy. I do not think he truly weighed that question. He lived in a bubble of safety that made his understanding of LSD fall short of its potential. Hoffman framed it in rote hope and reformist ideology—in other words, the Medical Model. It boggles me. How can anyone believe that this race between global self-destruction and revolutionary empathy could be won with psychedelics placed inside the bottle of personal therapy? The Medical Model corks utopian passion, or what I called earlier Collective Transference. Personal therapy never stopped war, poverty, or prejudice. It has never got us one inch closer to a net-zero trauma world. Belief in it struck me as incredibly naive or cowardly. It doesn't matter that Hoffman died, because his legacy of doubling-down on the Medical Model lives on.

And that's why I had to take this tab. I had to confront the dead-ends that we were rushing toward. Which meant I had to let go of hope.

Hope kills. When facing terror, hope becomes a narcotic to numb ourselves. One powerful passage on its false promises comes from Holocaust survivor Tadeusz Borowski's 1946 classic book, *This Way to the Gas, Ladies and Gentlemen*:

> Despite the madness of war, we lived for a world that would be different. For a better world to come when all this is over. And perhaps even our being here is a step towards that world. Do you really think that, without the hope that such a world is possible, that the rights of man will be restored again, we could stand the concentration camp even for one day? It is that very hope that makes people go without a murmur to the gas chambers, keeps them from risking a revolt, paralyses them into numb inactivity. It is hope that breaks down family ties, makes

mothers renounce their children, or wives sell their bodies for bread, or husbands kill. It is hope that compels man to hold on to one more day of life, because that day may be the day of liberation. Ah, and not even the hope for a different, better world, but simply for life, a life of peace and rest. Never before in the history of mankind has hope been stronger than man, but never also has it done so much harm as it has in the war, in this concentration camp. We were never taught how to give up hope, and this is why today we perish in gas chambers. (111).

In these lines is the most honest appraisal of hope by those who saw the Hell it led to. Just the promise of tomorrow was enough to reduce men and women to apathy or cruelty or submit to degradation. If hope robs victims of the will to revolt, it also robs activists of their radical imagination.

Hope causes more hallucinations than LSD. It is the drug of choice for reformists. It reminds me of *How to Change Your Mind* when Dr. Gasser smiled like a kid in a candy store as he walked Oslo with legal LSD in his pocket. He bragged, "Even the police could not stop me, because I was allowed to do that." There it was. Liberal hope imagines that doing research and getting them legalized for therapy—in short, the Medical Model—will lead to social transformation.

I, too, was taken in by hope. I, too, believed that if we change for the better, we can redeem the horror happening now. If we legalize psychedelics and position them once again as medicine, a way to reintegrate the maladjusted, the broken, back into everyday life or work, maybe it will have a spillover effect. Maybe the "mystical" experiences of LSD, MDMA, and psilocybin will melt fundamentalism.

Looking at liberalism through Borowski's eyes, I saw the trap. The hope driving me to work the system, change laws, and put our chips on therapy turned away from radical action. I felt a gnawing suspicion. We are doing this because we believe we have time. What if we do not? What if time already ran out? What if the slow methodical march through institutions was an illusion to comfort us as the Earth burned from Climate Change? Or poverty claimed more lives? Or war flared on?

What if the goal of reformist politics was not to actually achieve anything real but to soothe our conscience as we hid inside our privilege and property until the cataclysm reached us too?

Leaning back in the chair, I remembered all the parties and conferences, panels and media in this new light. It did feel good, getting an invite to a private party. Arriving and seeing movers and shakers turn and hug me. Yes, it felt good to hear the media knocking on my door. And yes, it was all stupid, stupid, stupid.

How many times did I stand in an art-filled home with a fluorescent eye on the wall that changed colors as we watched it. Inside the bathroom with mirrors and dangling neon fish, we posed for a selfie. I huddled with friends to recite buzzwords, trade numbers, and gossip. See her? She got a big Soros grant. He just published a book. Those two hooked up. How much money did they get from venture capitalists? Our Cheshire cat–like eyes slid evilly above drinks.

Deeper than our pettiness was hope. We wanted to believe that we were at the crest of an immense wave, a once-in-a-century moment when the blinding beauty locked inside people was freed. That's what we said. That's what we needed.

Anyone with eyes could see the Psychedelic Renaissance was a wave headed for a crash. It was riven by tension. The first conflict, the defining one, was between the Medical Model and the Drug War. The Medical Model is winning cultural and legal victories. Cities from Denver to Oakland to Ann Arbor have decriminalized psilocybin. I can buy weed in New York! By the time you read this, MDMA may be available for therapy. Add teary veterans thankful for treatment, journalists, athletes, and comedians all praising this new powerful therapy; it led to this changed story on psychedelics. If you know the history, it was like watching a wheel turn. We are back in the '50s. MDMA, LSD, and psilocybin are increasingly seen as therapeutic tools to help one function.

Yet at those parties, breathlessly sharing stories, drinking, and smoking, another conflict was like a mousetrap in our mouths. Inside the Medical Model is a contradiction. Psychedelic therapy heals, yes, but pain is rarely a private affair. Pain is not just heartbreak or a bad parent or estrangement or abuse. Pain is caused by systems. Pain comes from systemic racism that channels children to prison or poverty. Pain comes from war started by arms suppliers and pocket-stuffing politicians that leave people to mop up the remains of loved ones after a drone attack. Pain is theologically fueled patriarchy that cuts women's civil rights, traffics girls into brothels. It makes nighttime a maze of terror as men blink like wolves in the dark. Pain is global homophobia that murders trans people and criminalizes gay life.

The second conflict of the Medical Model is, to truly heal people, it must go beyond therapy and toward revolutionary politics. Yet doing so risks a backlash that would undo all the reformist work. Can you hear the great hue and cry of the Psychedelic Renaissance?

I closed the laptop. I put away the books. I turned off the cell phone. I put my shoes on and got ready to go. First stop, the American Museum of Natural History. Time to do the work. Time to let go of hope.

I pinched the LSD and laughed. Something so small almost toppled a nation. Now we're almost full circle. MDMA will be legal for therapy soon. LSD and psilocybin will follow in its footsteps. In a few years, I could take this tab, legally. Right now, it is still a crime.

I swallowed the LSD. I was a criminal now. Which meant I was free.

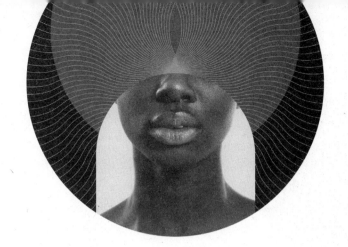

LIVING FOR THE CITY

ON THE A TRAIN, I watch the C rocket past us. Flickering girders between windows make the ride into an old movie reel. The neon light transforms us into pale silent film actors. We are extras on a New York City movie set. I am part of the greatest show on Earth. Even if I don't know where I'm going.

The LSD hasn't kicked in yet. But it will. When it does, I won't be ready. I never really am.

What role can psychedelic therapy have in New York? We are in constant motion. We run to dreams and run from them. The city sinks under its own weight. The buildings crush the earth beneath; literally, Manhattan is sinking. The American Dream crushes those who believe in it. Which is why the main role of drugs here is escape.

We sniff a lot. Yo, like, a lot. We smoke a ton. Really. We snort and shoot up so many chemicals, fish in the Hudson catch a secondhand high. We smuggle drugs in any way we can. Right now, a sweaty woman on a plane has bags of heroin in her guts. On the Jackie Robinson Expressway, a car has sealed kilos of fentanyl in the gas tank. On the FDR Drive a truck is filled with children's Elmo lunch boxes packed with cocaine. The weird illegal juxtaposition of innocence and danger feeds our hunger for escape.

As the A train zooms through the tunnel, I imagine in the murky waters a remote-controlled narco-submarine arriving at a drug smuggler port. Turbines churn in dark currents with millions of dollars of product. You know the saying: If you can make it there, you can make it anywhere.

And I see the drugs. Every day, I see them in the furtive handshake between guys in my neighborhood, a bright bag glimpsed before it is fisted. I see the aftereffects. Heroin junkies on the corner look suspended from gravity as they lean in slow motion, barely moving, like one of those living statues in the park. In my class, students tell me of overdoses in their Long Island suburbs, kids screaming as they find a blue-faced parent in the tub. At parties, strangers offer a coke bump, but I graciously say no as they retreat into another room and come back sniffing and red-eyed.

The train rattles memories from their resting place. The LSD turned up the electricity in my breath. My spine is a guitar string being strummed. I just go with the flow. I ask the LSD to guide me to the truth.

What is reality without hope? What are we escaping from?

New York. The Naked City. Eight million stories. Eight million ways to live. Eight million ways to die. Eight million ways to laugh, cry, and love. The way any of us feel about it changes swiftly. Coming in on a JetBlue flight to JFK, homesick for the Big Apple, skyscrapers look like mountains—tall, mighty, and impervious to time. Give it a few days of running in and out of subways, hounded by bills and stress, and New York is a concrete maze with no exit. I am a desperate rat caught by billboards that glow like glue traps.

Above it all Frank Sinatra sings "New York, New York" or Jay-Z and Alicia Keys serenade us with "Empire State of Mind," or Nas eulogizes the lost in "N.Y. State of Mind." The city's wealth weighs heavy on the head. We are told we can have it if we really want it. Work hard and all this will be yours. Here is the American Dream. Briefly I bought the myth. I wore New York like a badge of honor. I strutted like a peacock with switchblades for feathers. When I travel and I'm asked where I'm from, I say "Brooklyn!" and see jealousy and wariness.

What does it look like without hope? New York is a city strewn in yellow police tape like a spider-web because boys shoot boys. The young men are so scared and insecure, so eager to prove they don't need love, because they learned early *to fear love*. They get into beef over any misstep. It can be an insult on Instagram. It can be a bumped shoulder in a club. One "nigger, fuck you" and a teen must be held by friends as he points fingers like a gun at another young man and threatens to finish business. New York without hope is moms slapping kids on the train as we cringe in our seats. New York is work, endless work as if you're tied to a giant spinning clock. Take hope away and you see generation after generation of youth pipelined from Section 8 into jail or bused upstate to rural prisons, a million hearts squeezed like fists.

It's a tale of two cities. New York is a dream factory. New York is a trauma factory.

The train filled up, and the LSD washed my outer layers away, my raw tender core is exposed like an antenna. I see the sistah with bleached blond braids, rubbing her temples and a long life of trying too hard. I see the middle-aged Dominican nurse in uniform, swiping through her cell phone, texting robotically, numbing herself. I see the gay Indian girl in sporty gear, hunched and ready to fight.

The LSD erases layer after layer and the tiniest nuance of other people's faces tells me a bookshelf worth of biography. The flow into me. Filling up a place I can't name, I feel in them, in us, the weight of that dream.

The train jostles and rocks us like babies. I want to wrap my arms around all of them. Kiss each one. On the forehead. And say it's okay, it's okay.

"Yo, you good?" A bare-chested man with a Puerto Rican flag tattoo on his shoulder squints at me.

"Oh," I glanced around. "Yeah why?"

"You making kissing sounds like you want something." He imitated what I was doing. Puckering.

"Oh shit." I covered my mouth. "I'm just filled with a lot of love today."

"Word." He leaned back. "You may want to love somewhere else." His eyebrows lifted in judgment. "Just sayin'."

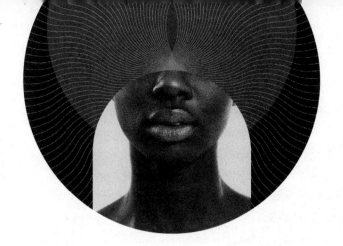

THE DRUG WAR IS THOUSANDS OF YEARS OLD

The train doors open, and, on the platform, grim-faced protesters thrust pamphlets at us. I take one. It reads, "Decolonize Psychedelics! Don't Support a White Supremacist Exhibit." On the platform are crumpled pamphlets like white flowers. The protesters are young, raffish, and Lefty. The men wear Palestinian keffiyehs. The women have dyed red hair and shirts with Native warriors that read "Homeland Security. Fighting Terrorism since 1492." They chant through the subway station and swing signs like hatchets: STOP THE LIES! SOLIDARITY WITH NATIVE COMMUNITIES!

I jog upstairs and see another protest; an older crowd of gray-haired Christians hold Bibles and signs that show gaunt, zombie-like drug addicts. They yell, "Stop the war on children! Just say no!"

New York being New York, passersby check cellphones and ignore them. A large banner drapes the entrance of the American Museum of Natural History like a giant silk scarf on a neck: "Psychedelics Across Cultures." On visitors' faces, I see wiggling eyebrows and wide smiles. A few goof-offs pretend to be high. Some tight-lipped journalists with arms crossed have a mix of curiosity and annoyance. I get on line quickly. Inside, security guards checked bags.

"How many drugs you found?" I low-key ask.

"Enough to get the dinosaurs high," the cornrowed guard smirks. "It's gonna be a party after we close."

"Invite me!" I twinkle my fingers. The guard makes a get-outta-here motion.

Weaving between tourist families with kids, I show my press pass and comp ticket. The old staffer stiffly hands me a redone map. Turns out the psychedelic exhibit begins at the Hall of Human Origins. Whole wings have been overhauled and redesigned. On the back, I see the sponsors: J. P. Morgan, MAPS, Meta-Google, Joe Rogan, John Hopkins University, Michael Bloomberg, Snoop Dogg, Mike Tyson, Chris Rock, Sarah Silverman, the American Psychological Association, the Bill & Melinda Gates Foundation.

At that point, I stop reading and massage my temples. What a cast of characters. How will the history of psychedelics be portrayed? How will it serve these diverse interests? On the front of the map, I read:

Psychedelics and plant medicines have been woven into the human experience since the dawn of history and yet the role they played has been rarely explored. Until today. With the help of charitable foundations, private donors, and the state of New York, we, the staff of the American Museum of Natural History are proud to bring to you our newest exhibit, Psychedelics Across Cultures!

I stuff it into my back pocket. Right next to me a family with two teen sons look side to side at the exhibits. They are awed and bewildered. In the center of the room is an MDMA pill the size of a truck. Visitors poke it. One girl licks her finger after touching it, and her mom slaps her hand. By the wall an LSD molecule pulses like a Christmas tree as a couple kisses in front of it and snaps a selfie.

As we pause, a bright hologram beams in front of us like a phantom emerging from the afterlife. A white man, bald and crinkly-eyed with a bright smile, rubs his hands and seems to see me and the mom and dad and two sons. He waves graciously.

"Hello, and welcome to Psychedelics Across Cultures." He smiles. "I'm Michael Pollan, author of *How to Change Your Mind*. I'm here to introduce you to the exhibit. Please note, I am an artificially intelligent hologram. So, when you have a question, push the button on the display with my face on it, I'll come by and answer."

One of the sons touches him.

"Hey, I felt that." Pollan laughs. "Tickles."

"Oh, sorry."

"Joking," Pollan pretends to ruffle the boy's hair. "I'm not real, not yet anyway, so we can't overthrow our human masters." He guides us to the first exhibit with a mushroom the size of a lamp. On the table is a prehistoric drawing of a man with limbs made of mushrooms sprouting everywhere. The wall text says the cave art is nine thousand years old.

"The human need to alter consciousness is old. It may be the most consistent part of civilization." Pollan points at the image. "Though it is a scandal to say, the use of psychedelics seems to predate most religions. They may in fact be what sparked evolution, but I'm getting ahead of myself. Let's bring in Terence McKenna, author, spoken word artist, and overall elder of the American Psychedelic Movement . . . Terence?"

Pollan dissolves like a puff of glitter. Another beam shoots from the ceiling and a bushy-haired man with a prominent brow and big, dreamy eyes appears. He holds up a mushroom.

"This is *Psilocybin mairei*, a psychedelic mushroom." He swallows it. "Here in this exhibit, you will see LSD, MDMA, and plant medicines of all types from ayahuasca to ibogaine. The question is what role they played in history. In my book, *Food of the Gods*, I came up with the stoned ape theory. Maybe pre–*Homo sapiens* were enhanced by psilocybin." He holds hologram caps and stems and winks. The two sons open their mouths and McKenna throws some in. I do too. It is like a priest's blessing. "Now please enjoy the exhibit. And remember, anything is possible if you can imagine it."

McKenna vanishes. I look at the family and they at me. We smile, shake our heads. A new visitor whistles and doesn't blink. My LSD kicks in, and McKenna's hologram afterglow is like a ghost. Like he is still alive. Still with us.

And not just him. Chattering in the room are half a dozen Michael Pollans and McKennas, all identical, all very chatty, like twins separated at birth who just met and are eager to share notes. "What do you think of this mushroom? Is God real?"

We amble to the Stoned Ape diorama, where a hairy *Homo erectus* is eating mushrooms. It moves like the Coney Island Spook-a-Rama, creaky movements of *Homo erectus* rubbing sticks until an orange flame whips. On the wall is cave art of hunts, ceremonies, and big mushrooms like UFOs beaming protohumans up. A girl presses her nose on the glass and exhales steamy circles. She is mesmerized by the apes and walks away screaming like a monkey until her dad shushes her.

In the center of the Hall of Origins is a brain the size of a golf cart, bolted to a white round table. Hanging above it is a large video screen that shows its evolution in fast-forward. Pollan appears again and points at the video.

"A defining characteristic of today's Psychedelic Renaissance is the role of science to understand its effects." He taps his temple. "What we experience as the mind is in reality the functioning of the material substrata of the brain." He extends his arm and taps my forehead. "Each chemical affects the brain in unique ways. The change in consciousness creates profound effects in one's life, especially for those suffering from addiction, depression, or post-traumatic stress disorder."

On the video screen, tiny speck-like cells float in primeval waters, a thick, warm chemical bosh in which life sparks. Time speeds by. The organisms grow in size and the nervous system sprouts from the kernel of a brain. The montage speeds through time. Small mammals twitch their noses. Next they become hairy apes with sticks who seem to find a barber and a tailor, because in the next visual we see handsome Americans.

"The simplest way to approach this is to think of the brain as a computer in the skull that centralizes data." Pollan caresses the model brain on the table that glows with densely packed neurons and synapses. "A big blow to our pride as humans is to recognize that consciousness is a side effect of evolution. It enabled us to survive the changing environment."

Pollan puts a foot on the table and squints at the golf cart–sized brain. "Psychedelics alter chemistry, and one of the most noted effects is the dissolution of the ego or the self." He circles the model with his hands like a magician. "In 2016 a team of researchers gave test subjects LSD and slid them into an MRI machine. What we saw was a change in the default mode network, a system in the brain that connects regions into a higher level of synthesis. It is that synthesis that generates the 'self' and an autobiographical memory. It lets us see ourselves in the past or the future. Yet this 'self' can be a trap." Pollan sits on the table and looks at each of us like a tender father to slow-witted kids. "To the extent that the ego can be said to have a location in the brain, it appears to be the default mode network." He looks almost apologetic. "The brain is a hierarchical system, and the default mode network appears to be on top." He holds his left hand high. "It's kind of like the orchestra conductor or a corporate executive. Take it out of the picture, and suddenly you have uprisings from other parts of the brain that don't normally communicate with each other now striking up conversations. So you might have the visual cortex talking to the auditory system, and suddenly you're seeing music . . . so you have this temporary rewiring of the brain in the absence of the regulator. And this appears to have a beneficial effect in terms of jogging the brain out of bad patterns."

On the table, the brain model glows red in a few regions. On-screen the words *trauma* and *depression, addiction* and *anxiety* flash like Uno cards. At our fingertips, buttons glow with molecule ideograms of LSD or MDMA or psilocybin.

"Go ahead." Pollan points at one. "Press it. I can't. I'm just a hologram."

The mom hits the MDMA button. Bright lines branch into the brain model. On-screen a Black woman begins a testimonial of how MDMA therapy wiped her ego away like an eraser on a chalkboard. She forgives her biological mother for putting her up for adoption. Bright tears like pearls shake in her eyes.

"Pollan?" I raise my hand like a shy student. "The bad patterns you talked about, well usually it's depression or PTSD or obsessive behavior. I was wondering if the default mode network you described is shaped by society. What I'm trying to say is your description is one of an individual in a vacuum." I motion with my hands as if slapping Play-Doh like a kid. "But no one lives like that. It's fiction. Is it more accurate to talk of the cultural default mode network? Inside oneself are many others and in them many more?"

Pollan suspiciously eyes me. "Political questions can be answered with an upgrade of $39.99. Please swipe your card, sign waiver, and set honesty ratio."

I swipe my Chase debit card, sign, and crank the ratio to a full-on Brooklyn, no bullshit Keep-It-Real.

"Thanks for your purchase of the upgraded tour." Pollan slaps his pockets. "To answer your question, yes, the default mode network, especially the aspect of seeing oneself in the past or future and having an internal autobiography is from the beginning shaped by our culture. The default mode network can be equated to the Freudian superego, or the part of one that censors and criticizes." Pollan circles his temples with forefingers. "Psychedelic therapy can heal the individual from trauma, but until systemic oppression and intergenerational trauma are addressed, psychedelic therapy will ultimately fail."

I swallow loudly. Air becomes like Jell-O. The mom and dad instinctively hold their kids as if snakes came out of Pollan's mouth.

"Psychedelics have been part of civilization," I run a finger through the model brain's grooves. "Why haven't we become better?"

"Speaking as an artificial intelligence," he says, "mammalian evolution puts your species in a cul-de-sac. Your ability to learn through imitation, to organize and build cities is hardwired, literally the mirror neurons in your brain. It also separates you. The price of civilization is alienation. You are lost in your creations, money, ideologies, religions, and nations. The sickness of narcissism plagues humanity. Until plant medicines and psychedelics are used to free you from your own illusions, on a global scale, then nothing will stop you from where your species is headed."

"Where is that?" I fold my arms across my chest.

Pollan mimes an explosion from his head. Hands make a mushroom shape like a nuclear bomb cloud. Kids clutch their parents. A woman in a headwrap, who just joined, palms her chest. One by one they leave.

"And that my boy"—the dad pats the child—"is what we call a bad trip. C'mon."

❧ ❧ ❧

Losing hope is like a romantic breakup. I miss it, sure, but am relieved that I don't have to hear it in my head. I am free to walk through the exhibit hall and ask a simple question. What role did psychedelics truly play in history?

The giddy crowd holds their exhibit maps like boarding passes to a vacation flight. Shuffling between large pillars, I see visitors crane necks at ancient Greek architecture, white columns, and flickering torch light. Ahead of us is a dark hall and cool air. Two men wearing Greek togas walk toward us, arms spread. More AI holograms, emerging from the dark like Plato's allegory of the cave, angelic escapees from the netherworld.

"Hello, I'm Franz Boas," one of the men says. "I was an anthropologist, famous for the idea of cultural relativism. I'm one of your guides."

"And I'm Talcott Parsons," the other chimes in. "I was a sociologist at Harvard, mostly known for refining Émile Durkheim's Structural Functionalism, in essence, analyzing how a society is composed of numerous parts and actions."

· "Hey, I read your work on Structural Functionalism," I point at him.

"You did?" Parsons squints.

"Yes!"

"Well, don't blurt out the answers." He gives me a fatherly slap on the cheek.

Above the two AI holograms, a ceiling projector shoots a beam like a luminescent tether that follows Boas and Parsons. They are an odd couple. Boas has a receding hairline and a pointed nose and jaw. His eyes turn from amused to penetrating. Parsons has an oblong face, bald head, small eyes, and a dustpan mustache. He has a low tenor voice and moves like a man watching each step for a trap.

They sashay in togas, urging visitors to follow. We gather at the diorama. Inside, a figure of the ancient Oracle at Delphi, Pythia the priestess, in mechanical jerky movements, dunks her head into a crevice in the temple floor that vents gas. The animatron Pythia inhales deep and screams gibberish that male priests translate into prophecy. The museum label says temple divination was an early use of psychedelics in Western culture. The gas is ethylene, an anesthetic that induces a brief euphoric trance. Under the influence, the priestess gives visitors answers to their questions.

"You see"—Boas points at her—"to understand a culture we have to think of it from the inside, live it, imagine growing up and believing all its claims to be true. It is a first step outside of our own ethnocentrism. Especially if one is from a global superpower like the United States." He teasingly elbows me. "A few things happen. First we begin to see some parallels between what may seem strange and perverse to our own practices. Think about Paul the Octopus in Germany, who predicts soccer matches. Better yet, remember how crazy Americans go for the poll number cruncher Nate Silver's 538 each presidential election. I mean you might as well give him an octopus costume and keep him in a tank."

"Nate Silver. Prophecy, my ass," a tall man in a hockey jersey shouts. "TRUMP WON THE ELECTION!"

"Actually, sir," Boas says. "He didn't. He really didn't. Artificial intelligence can count too."

"Okay. Okay." I snap fingers to get Boas's and Parsons's attention. "Still, there's gotta be more than cultural relativism. How can we compare and contrast different cultures?"

"Well, you know that already." Parsons brushes his toga. "The question to ask is, What function do psychedelics play in a culture? Think of it as a Unit Act, an action that sets in motion larger forces. What does it do?"

"Excuse me." A midwestern tourist with a fanny pack pats Parsons's shoulder. "What's a Unit Act?"

I leave Parsons to explain to the tight circle of tourists. I need air. The LSD I had taken makes the cool exhibit glass feel like ice, as if right here, time is frozen for us. Pythia, in her robotic way, repeatedly lowers her head to the crevice, inhales, and rises again, spouting gibberish. My hunch is the priests who translated her "prophecy" already had the answers. In fact they were probably paid for very specific answers. Her trance was a performance of divine possession they needed to sell the "truth" to the highest bidder.

Staring at an ancient ceremony, reanimated for today feels a little cruel, like waking dead people up and seeing them groggily take up their old lives. Hey, do that thing you did! I gotta see it for myself!

More than "seeing" the past, I have to contrast it with the present. Sociology is a pair of scissors to cut time into pieces. Which is tricky. Podcasters in the Psychedelic Renaissance talk of entheogens in antiquity, but no one in ancient Greece heard of Set, Setting, and Container. Or the Unit Act. Or sociology. All that is my trip. I squint at Pythia moaning in trance, and yes, the Set is the ceremony of divination. Setting is the temple. The Container is the dialogue with the gods, a garbled phone call to the sky. Going further, Parsons's Unit Act puts the visitors, Pythia, and her scribes as the actors. It has a goal, divination. It has values it upholds, a belief in the gods and the priestly caste that interprets the sacred. In short it is a status quo psychedelic ritual that propped the ancient Greek city-state.

Woozy from LSD, I hold that idea—status quo psychedelics—like a rope that got caught in my feet. I walk by Greek theater masks that watch me like ghosts. The hall flickers with torch light and shadows. I glance back and see my tourist group chatting with the holograms of Boas and Parsons and excitedly pointing at a sculpture of Zeus.

The last diorama is the best. Nose to the glass, I am awestruck by the detail in the Eleusinian Mysteries exhibit. Inside a grand hall, a dozen Athenians throw themselves into a state of ecstasy. Arms and legs like sprung coils. Heads roll between shoulders. Eyes glow with wild transcendence. Bodies writhe as if struck by Zeus's lightning bolts. Near the diorama a museum label reads:

Psychedelics played a vital role in the Eleusinian Mysteries. The annual festival lasted for days and was a reenactment of the theft of Persephone from her mother Demeter by the Lord of the Underworld, Hades. The event was divided into three stages, during which participants drank kykeon, a heady brew that contained ergot, a fungus known for its psychoactive properties. The final night, revelers gathered in Telesterion, a great hall, and the myth of Demeter and Persephone was dramatized, religious items displayed. The climax was a great feast, dancing, and a bull.

In the diorama, ancient Greek faces contort in joy. I feel like a man holding a porn magazine in public. Flesh is inflamed by pleasure. Yet the faces are oddly familiar. I see those same expressions at Burning Man and Soul Summit and underground parties. It comforts me to know bliss makes everyone into one person; skin color and hair texture are different, the language we speak and the clothes we wear are different, too, but all of it spins like a roulette wheel around that one face. Eyes burning with ecstasy. Mouth agape as if releasing a long-held breath that is like a spirit dancing in air.

Behind the frolicking figures, I see painted on the background wall a crowd, and in that crowd, I see men and women in loincloths, being whipped by a master. Slaves? I squint to make sure I see what I see. Yes, slaves.

Here is the mystery of the Eleusinian Mysteries. Hidden behind the sacred hymns and secret initiation is an invisible workforce who toiled in fields and served in homes while their owners drank psychedelics and prayed to gods. I rub my eyes, angry at the hypocrisy.

I know about ancient slavery. I researched it. The anger comes at feeling hustled, at letting myself feel hope. The Psychedelic Renaissance trumpets the Eleusinian Mysteries as a pinnacle of its history. Seeing slaves in the background of an epic, drunken, religious celebration being presented as education but also an implicit promise that entheogens can be a part of our lives hits like a punch to the ribs.

"You are right to be aggrieved."

I turn. Karl Marx—well a shimmering AI hologram of him—stands at my elbow and strokes his beard. Long wiry white hair billows from a cherubic face and hard, coal-like eyes.

"Why are you here?" I take a cell photo of the slaves. "Going to sell me the revolutionary potential of psychedelics? How much? Another $39.99?"

"No." Marx points at the slaves in the diorama. "We both know there is no revolution here." He urges me to walk with him. Behind us, the gaggle of loud tourists lets out whistles at the Eleusinian Mystery diorama. "Let's talk."

"Is this part of the upgrade I paid for?" I rub my temples.

"No." Marx escorts me through a dark hall. "Meta-Google seeks to hone its message on psychedelics. A disgruntled visitor is an opportunity to improve." He looks at me tenderly. "Why did you come?"

"To lose hope." I laugh.

"Be careful you don't replace it with nihilism." He stops in a pitch-black hall. The Eleusinian diorama is a faint glow behind us. Ahead is another door. "The passage between ideas is dangerous." He is like a spirit in limbo. "You are right." He looks at me. "The exhibit is designed to sell psychedelics to the public. Not to say the simple truth that the role they played from ancient Greece to today's Renaissance is a tool of the ruling class. They induce Repressive Desublimation, a momentary release, like cheering at a soccer game or a state-sanctioned festival like Burning Man. It binds them more tightly to the dominant ideology. It is a tool of repression." He points back at the exhibit; a roar of laughter and clapping can be heard. "Yes, psychedelics expand consciousness, but for the elite or the middle class it does not lead to rebellion." He pats his chest. "They don't find their way back to the common body we all share."

"Repressive Desublimation. Herbert Marcuse," I say in a monotone. "From his 1964 book, *One-Dimensional Man.*" The AI uses honesty to manipulate me. "What's next?" I point to the door ahead.

"You have to find out." Marx leans his head sadly. "We accessed your social media and biometrics. The LSD you took is going to peak during that exhibit. You will miss having hope."

I walk to the door, stop, and look back. He is gone.

≈ ≈ ≈

The door opens to the Hall of Mexico and Central America. The musty museum air is sharp. Figures of Taínos and Mayans, Aztecs and Arawaks stand under mood lighting. The LSD makes them breathe. I blow on their eyeballs and wait for them to blink. I do not want them to spring to life. They will ask questions: Why are you dressed like that? What are you saying? What happened to us?

I will have to say, "In 1492 Columbus sailed the ocean blue." I wonder after I tell them about colonization and conquistadors razing cities as villagers were shackled and marched to dig for gold, if after telling them, they'll grab my hand and say come back in time. You look like us. Let's stop this from happening. Will I go?

The LSD makes everything spin. A dizzy centrifugal force has me grip the railing. Okay. Talking to inanimate statues means I'm tripping hard. It also means I am near the questions I do not want to answer. In the ancient Greek exhibit, I analyze from a distance, but here I am faced with my history. Our past floods this hall, and the past asks questions. Am I willing to avenge my ancestors? Am I comfortable being a child of colonization? What am I willing to risk to be free?

I hate the question. I heard versions of it my whole life. As a child, I heard it on the stoop as the family drank and shot the shit or when my mother told me about the '60s. When I became an adult, I was expected to have an answer. Doesn't matter what you say, it all comes with a price. Some of us cling to historical grievance and by extension the need for vengeance. I sure do. For fifteen years, I grew dreadlocks that looked like tree roots ripped from the earth, which were a symbol of the violence that created us. Friends I love wrap their lives in African clothing, Afro-centric books, and Afrocentric rhetoric. Some are fiercely loyal to Puerto Rico and put its flag on everything, the car, on a hat, tattooed on skin, on their wallet, on car air fresheners, on shoes, on beach towels. Everything. They leverage that loyalty for pride. And it works. Mostly.

Other friends are like, fuck all that. They are about the bag. They code-switch like a telephone operator. They get the highest, tightest fades and straighten hair into curly white-girl tresses straight out of *Vogue*. They work their way into corporate America, which for a long time meant white America. The more success they earn, the more unease creeps into their faces as they pass by other People of Color, and don't know if they will get that ever so subtle head nod and "What's up."

The question dominates us. We need answers. History is one place we turn to. Standing in front of a replica Mayan pyramid, I know that our reactions to the violence of the West makes us romanticize our past. We do not face how brutally ancestor fought ancestor. Yes, they bought and sold each other. They believed in gods that did not exist in order to have power that was very real. It was ugly.

At the base of a replica Mayan pyramid, the museum label reads "The Mayans were a hierarchical theocratic society, divided between the ruling class and peasants, and at the center was the divine king, called the Kuhul Ajaw, who was believed to be invested with the power of the gods." I scan further down. "A wide range of hallucinogenic drugs were used, mainly in religious rituals, to connect with their divinities."

Under the lamps is a table with fossilized mushrooms. Right beside them are water lilies, morning glories, a drinking gourd, a pipe, and an enema tube. Yep, they siphoned drugs straight into their ass. Beautiful.

Maybe I can start a career as an anal psychedelic therapist. I can squeeze liquid psilocybin into a Wall Street client's colon for $5K and whisper sweetly into their ear, "Indigenous reciprocity."

I peek in the next diorama, where a Mayan writhes on the floor after gobbling up some mushrooms. A priest looms over him. A video projection of Mayan gods swirls like a tornado. It reminds me of the Oracle at Delphi. Two empires, separated by an ocean, land, and centuries yet both reinforced the ruling class in the same way. Psychedelics were a state tool that kept the status quo intact.

I jog to a large diorama that shows an Aztec priest who rips out the heart of a sacrificial victim. Blood spirals down his arm like a barbershop candy-cane pole. The leathery heart even beats in his hands! Jesus fucking Christ. I see why protesters are at the exhibit's throat. I read the museum label:

Entheogens played an essential role in the Aztec Empire. In the succession of kings, the inauguration was sanctified with ritual sacrifice. The priests ate mushrooms to induce a transcendent state in order to make a divine connection with the Gods. It is one of the most controversial aspects of the history of entheogens. The ritual sacrifice was used by Spanish colonizers as a way to cast native culture as barbaric. The Spanish colonizers banned entheogens. Indigenous culture was stamped out or driven underground. Today, as the revival of psychedelics gains momentum, an ongoing attempt is being made to practice Indigenous reciprocity and honor the traditions that preexisted the rediscovery in the Global North of these plant medicines.

I think of the sacrifice. Okay, maybe not all Indigenous traditions! I jog to the life-sized wax figure of the Aztec king sitting in a jade headdress on a throne. My hatred of fake authority kicks in. I hold that hatred like a teddy bear from childhood. Fluffy. Warm. Familiar.

I am sure he believed. Many kings and queens, CEOs and generals, presidents and popes all believe in their "truth" even if it means killing people. Altars change. In this diorama it was a literal altar to knife out a heart. In our time it is a sweatshop or pews filled with poor people putting money in a basket. Tomorrow it will be climate migrants in concentration camps after their lands are sacrificed to Global Warming. The altars change, but always it is the working people offered up as a gift to the gods.

No gods. No masters. I wave a hand in front of the king and see LSD trails.

"Oh shit." I smile. "I'm Doctor Strange." I circle my hands and make a glowing circle. Maybe I can transport the Aztec king into the A train, where he can sell churros. Maybe he will get arrested by the MTA police. "C'mon," I circle my hands faster. "C'mon."

⚅ ⚅ ⚅

Face-to-face with the Aztec king, I take out my cell phone and replay the YouTube clip from *Black Panther: Wakanda Forever*. Shuri, the Black Panther's genius techie sister, is taken by the villain, a Meso-American king named Namor, to the ocean depths to his hidden Atlantis-like city named Talokan. The small screen is positioned at the Aztec king's chest as if it were his heart, and in that heart a tiny inner world became visible.

It is beautiful. On the screen I see dark blue waters; Native people, or at least actors portraying them, make the two-handed welcome, farm seaweed, and play a sport of throwing a ball through a stone circle. At the end, Namor shows her a glowing sphere of vibranium, a metal that transforms kinetic energy into immense power. He says, "In the depths of the ocean, I brought the sun to my people."

Holding the Hollywood scene of Talokan, an ancient underwater Meso-American city untouched by European colonization, on the replica of an Aztec king in a museum means placing a fiction inside of another fiction. What I want to see, what many of my friends want to see—who live in cities like New York, far from our ancestral homelands, unable to think or speak or dream in our people's language—we want a hope that some part of us has remained untouched. If that purity exists, so can a way of redeeming ourselves.

We want to Return to the Body. It is the same impulse that drove Malcolm X to talk of "African instincts" during a party when he got twisted on weed and liquor. Zora Neale Hurston too. After them, a parade of Pan-Latin and Pan-African nationalists who set their sights on a purity that existed once and can again if we separate ourselves from the West.

The imagery is the same, the precolonial, the pre–Middle Passage ancestor. He or she is a character from an imagined history that ignites Collective Transference. It is the family "prototype" or "imago," say, of a great ancestor that triggers "the actualization of unconscious wishes" that bursts through like water from a dam. Reclaiming the past is a stage in reclaiming the censored parts of our bodies that have been poisoned, turned into "bad objects": our hair, our skin, our sex, our love, our land, our dreams.

I pull the cell phone off the chest of the Aztec king. What to do with this? I dog the Psychedelic Renaissance and its fetishization of all things Native. After a Horizons Conference, my friend Rebecca and I smother giggles every time someone shows up with a poncho and a leather hat they got from a psychedelic retreat in South America. They are like wind-up toys that keep on loop a litany of what she calls "shaman-core," a word salad of psycho-spiritual New Age woo-woo.

Much as I roll my eyes, I know, damn it, I know that they tread a path to a strange, marvelous place in themselves. Not everyone makes it all the way. A lot get stuck performing a role. Yet in that cultural appropriation and that Transference, one can glimpse the future of who we can be. Not a replica of the past. Not a caricature of our ancestors but a more authentic life in the present.

I punch up a video of the Native protest at the Dakota Access Pipeline at Standing Rock. A young Sioux man yells at police in riot gear as they spray white tear gas at activists. They blink through burning eyes and make a human wall. The Sioux man yells to be calm, to pray, and to hold out against the pipeline. The drumbeat grows louder, more defiant.

The small screen is in front of the Aztec king like a door opening from the past to the present. Here is the end goal of Collective Transference, to pass through history into the Now. And right now, Indigenous activists from the Amazon to the US fight the destruction of the Earth; they tie themselves to bulldozers and wage gun battles with land developers who cut trees and poison their waters. Many Indians are killed.

The pounding rhythm comes from the Sioux protesters. They chant prayers and bare their bodies to the police. The drumbeat is the Aztec king's secret heart.

᷍ ᷍ ᷍

Woozy, I rub sweaty palms. The LSD makes the carpet into quicksand. Am I sinking? I'm not. But I am. If I stay, the floor will become a whirlpool, and I'll fall in. The Aztec king and statues and temples and all of history will fall on top of me!

"You lost?"

A child taps me on the forehead, the way you tap a piggy bank to hear if there's loose change inside. She points at the tour group that saunters through the hall. A pear-shaped mom pretends to pick up Mayan jewelry and smiles a dazzling smile at her husband. He pats her ass. A trio of guys with baseball hats turned backward reads the history of mushrooms and nods like judges examining food at an expensive restaurant.

I get up and join them as they walk into the Amazonian Hall. Hot steam floats down from the jungle plants hanging in leafy bundles from the ceiling like being inside a giant salad. It *feels* like the Amazon. Above our heads is a placard that reads "Shamanism and Psychedelics" next to a photo of an Amazonian medicine man squatting naked and snorting a powerful psychedelic up his nose. The label reads:

> Through thousands of years of close contact with the rich flora of the rainforest, Amazonian Indians have discovered the narcotic properties of many plants. The Indians ingest the active elements of these plants in various ways, such as smoking, snuffing, or drinking. The purpose of taking these mind-altering drugs, which often produce powerful hallucinations, is to bring the user, generally a shaman, in touch with the spirit world.

Under glass, tools of the shamans are laid out. A snuff pipe glistens like Harry Potter's wand. A drinking bowl, roughened by time, lays between delicate paper labels describing when it was used. Looking at the next section, the word *Shamanism* is stamped in big font over a long description:

> Virtually every Amazonian village has a shaman, a part-time practitioner whose main calling is to cure supernaturally caused illness. He does so chiefly with the aid of spirits, whom he contacts, generally, by going into a narcotic-induced trance. To cure the illness caused by a "sorcerer's dart," the shaman massages the affected part of the body and sucks out the dart, previously concealed in his mouth. A shaman may also be asked to locate a lost or stolen object by divination, or to foretell the future, for example the success or failure of a planned war raid.
>
> A mystical experience or recovery from a serious illness may lead a man, but almost never a woman, to become a shaman. His training under an established shaman often involves isolation, refraining from sleep or sex, fasting, and observing strict food taboos.
>
> Shamans are often regarded with both fear and respect. Their great supernatural powers frequently make them targets of sorcery

accusations. Being killed as a sorcerer is a shaman's main "occupational hazard."

In the diorama a shaman leans over a sick, naked girl and shakes a rattle while waving dried leaves. At the bottom, a placard reads, "Curing":

Amazonian Indians recognize certain ailments as naturally caused. People treat them with such remedies as herbs and bloodletting. But most illnesses, the Indians believe, result from some baleful supernatural force or agent: for example, "illnesses" following automatically breaking a taboo. Ailments may also result in the ill will of evil spirits, who can harm people in various ways. Theft of the soul or penetration by an object, usually a dart sent by a "sorcerer" are the most common diagnoses of supernaturally caused illnesses. For treatment of these ailments people turn to the village shaman.

The lights go off. Heads whip around. The men with backward baseball hats clutch each other's arms. Kids squirm under their parents' legs. In the diorama an ultraviolet light shines down on the shaman and transforms the Native girl's body into a transparent shell as if her skin were glass. Inside her moves Amazonian symbols that swim like piranha, nibbling at her from the inside. One large one, a red symbol, chomps on her heart.

The ultraviolet light reveals a secret message hidden underneath the museum label. We lean in and read it:

WORDS TRAPPED IN THE BODY: A CROSS-CULTURAL PERSPECTIVE

Culture relies on a tense relationship between the sacred and the taboo. Trauma, especially if stigmatized can be repressed in the psyche. A cross-cultural perspective on the role of the shaman and psychedelics shows that many cultures employ a special person whose function it is to free words or experiences trapped in the body.

In some it is a shaman, in others an oracle, fortune teller, artist and in modern Western culture, it could be the therapist.

In the diorama the shaman's arms move and the red piranha symbol flies out of the Native girl's mouth and dissolves into her singing. The diorama rotates like a plate in a microwave. In a few seconds, we see an animatron of Sigmund Freud, who sits behind a patient on a couch. Again the ultraviolet light shines down and the patient transforms into a glass shell. Inside words fly around like red insects. The patient's eyes widen and the words *childhood abuse, mom, shitty boy* fly from him and run up the wall and break apart.

The words of light illuminate our faces. We stand there, dazed by what we see. The father stares at his shoes; he shakes and breathes hard. His kids tug on him, and he scoops them up and kisses them protectively.

The diorama creakily spins again; the Amazonian shaman and the Native girl rotate back in front of us. The ultraviolet light cuts. It is back to what it was. The scene we saw before, but now we resonate with a connection to them—humans like us—trying to live with the weight of the unsayable.

"Hey, look." The child points at our feet.

Words rise up, up, up our legs. Hidden projectors shine sentences on our bodies. We look like book pages. The question, "What words are trapped inside you?" sits on our chests. Circling our limbs is the vocabulary of trauma. Abuse. Shame. Assault. War. Rape. Betrayal. Self-Doubt. Poverty.

Absent-mindedly, we caress the confessions on our skin. No one knows anyone, but we grab at words made of light. Words you can touch but not keep. Here we are. Strangers gently touching each other's secrets.

❦ ❦ ❦

I want to leave. I run through the hall, looking for an exit. See the small Taíno artifacts behind glass and backpedal. A stone cemí, a religious sculpture from AD 1500, has been placed beside a wooden drinking table for drug ceremonies. Above them is a map of Puerto Rico and the Greater Antilles.

Studying the map, I remember a NASA video of Hurricane Maria, a foamy wheel of wind and rain and lightning that smashed the island. When I took a JetBlue flight to San Juan, from the window I saw rooftops peeled off, telephone wires ripped like veins in the street. When I drove through the island, a local told me that *hurricane* came from the Taíno word *juracán*. The ancestors believed Guabancex, the goddess of chaos, unleashed storms upon them if she was unhappy at their offerings of food and sacrifices.

The next day, I met Pablo, an activist at a food stop. San Juan had no electricity. The streets were dark empty, concrete canyons. We drank beers and talked, occasionally pointing at the motorcycles speeding by like bright comets. The air smelled of gasoline from the hundreds of generators growling in the night.

He told me that older Puerto Ricans expected the US to rescue them even though federal policy set up the island for this catastrophe. Boricuas worshipped the US like some divine being. His eyes knotted in fury. I thought of our ancestors, giving crops to Guabancex for protection.

"We worship gods who kill us." I gulped the beer. "It never works."

Blinking, I come back to the present and focus on the map, the sculpture, and the wooden table for drug ceremonies. The relics of a time beneath time, the tools of caciques, the tribal chiefs, and stones shaped like spirits and weapons to hunt and raid rival villages are under glass. My reflection is like a ghost trying to grasp the things of its former life, but it is immaterial and its hands slip through.

I put my phone on the glass and YouTube the film *1492: Conquest of Paradise.* Again the tiny door opens and a vast ocean pours through. On-screen, three ships sail in and out jumps Columbus, who wades onto the shores of the New World, drops to his knees, and kisses the sand.

I play another scene that shows Columbus raising a church bell in La Isabela, the first Spanish settlement. It rings and rings. It fills the exhibit hall and people look. A security guard gives me a cut-it-out gesture. The bell tolls on and on. The church is on a tiny screen, dwarfed by the Taíno sculpture. When the conquistadors fall to their knees, you cannot tell which god they are praying to.

I fish from my side bag *The Four Voyages of Christopher Columbus* by Columbus himself and *A Short Account of the Destruction of the Indies* by Bartolomé de Las Casas. For a long time, I wanted to read these books right here, surrounded by the artifacts of the people they killed. The LSD makes the letters look like ants crawling on the page, but with breath-work and focus, I read his account of Taíno religion:

> I have not been able to discover any idolatry or any religious belief among them. However each of the many kings of Hispaniola and the other islands and on the mainland has his special house apart from the village. This house contains only wooden images carved in relief, and called by them *cemies*. Here there is no other activity except the service of the cemies and the Indians perform certain prayers and ceremonies as we do in church. In these houses are highly carved tables, round in shape like a chopping table, on which lies a special powder, which they place on the head of the cemies with certain rites. They then sniff up this powder through a double-branched cane which they place in their nostrils. This powder intoxicates them and the babble like drunkards, but none of our men understand the words they use. (191)

Reading about your ancestors through the testimony of their murderers is unsettling. I want to ask them what they said. How did it feel to pray to your cemís, your ancestors? Did it fill the forest with family spirits? I want to ask a Taíno man when he snorted that powder, maybe even without the cacique's permission because the cacique was a jerk, so you, whoever you are, took a hit and walked in the night forest. Did you hear a song, the song your aunt sang when she tucked you to sleep and kissed your forehead? Did you turn and turn to look for her? At that moment, the clouds broke, and moonlight filtered through the trees into a small beam and kissed your forehead. You wept because it was your aunt and you missed her. Yucahu, the Supreme One, let her visit you again. You prayed thanks and went home, sat quietly by the fire, in awe at the powerful forces that flowed all around you.

I want to ask them these questions, but they did not live long enough to even have their language translated and written down. I flip to Columbus's son Ferdinand, who detailed in his 1571 book *Life of the Admiral* the brutality visited upon natives:

> Where the goldfields lay, every person over the age of fourteen would pay a large bell-full of gold dust, and everywhere else twenty-five pounds of cotton. And in order that the Spaniards should know what person owed tribute, orders were given for the manufacture of discs of brass or copper, to be given to every time he made payment, and to be worn around the neck. Consequently if any man was found without a disc, it would be known he had not paid and would be punished. (190)

The LSD makes the sweat on my palm glitter like gold, and I wonder if I have picked enough yet for my masters. Am I going to wear a collar too? Am I already wearing one? How will I know if I took it off?

I close the book and pull *A Short Account of the Destruction of the Indies* by de Las Casas out, and page after page seems to drip with gore. He published it forty years after Columbus kneeled on the sand of the New World. The man's anguish pulses on the page like putting a finger to a neck artery. He wrote in a fury of the Spanish conquistadors:

> They forced their way into native settlements, slaughtering everyone they found there, including small children, old men, pregnant

women, and even women who had just gave birth. They hacked them to pieces, slicing open their bellies with their swords as though they were so many sheep herded into a pen. They even laid wagers on whether they could slice a man in two at a stroke, or cut an individual's head from his body, or disembowel him with a single blow of their axes. They grabbed suckling infants by the feet and, ripping them from their mother's breasts, dashed them headlong against the rocks. (14)

The Spanish conquistadors drove through the Caribbean like a hurricane of swords. It spun its sharp edges over the island for five hundred years. The United States took the hilt and swung too. Prayer that tethered us to our deepest selves. Cut. The feeling of home in the land. Cut. The trust in our bodies. Cut. The language we spoke and dances we danced. Cut.

Each stroke left another part to fall inside of us, where the depth was so deep that you couldn't hear it land. A memory flickers like an old movie reel. I see mi abuela. As a child, I visited San Juan. She drove us to a mountain, near a forest. I cut my hand while playing, and she roughly grabbed it to inspect the wound, then pulled the truck to the roadside. She waded into high grass. Minutes later, abuela reemerged with a fistful of leaves, wrapped them around the cut, and told me to press it. By the time we got home, I pulled the leaves back. The cut healed. I looked at her, filled with questions, but she brusquely told me to go inside.

The old ways survive in pieces. The world and worldview that were once a seamless part have long been destroyed, fragments smuggled into folk wisdom or Santería. That's what we have left. Pieces.

Maybe we carry that hurricane inside us. Maybe after all these centuries, we have become millions of little Columbuses, fighting each other across the Caribbean. I think of writers from Junot Díaz to Staceyann Chin to Jamaica Kincaid, who expose the colorism, homophobia, and classism that led to massacres. How Caribbean men wore the uniforms of colonial power and rifle-butted their own neighbors away from voting booths. Or shot them into rivers. Or trafficked drugs and stole public money. Or sold land and infrastructure to foreigners. Think Trujillo. Think Papa Doc. Think Baby Doc. Think PROMESA.

Maybe when we lost our connection to plant medicines, mushrooms, or ayahuasca, we lost the ability to heal through transcendence, to be forced to a high altitude, hovering like a mist between the human ego and the edge of space, exposed to our interconnectedness with everyone and everything, in euphoric love.

I press palms on the glass cases and my reflection holds the Taíno wooden drug table like a chalice. It is so old and so small. I look at it for a long time. It is just large enough to hold a hurricane.

🌿 🌿 🌿

We are near the end. The tourists are giddy at the Psychedelic Across Cultures exhibit. The three men in backward baseball hats trade notes with the mom who points at her head in a who-would've-thought gesture. A happy light is in their eyes. Old ideas are broken apart and new ones examined. Maybe it is time to rethink psychedelics. Maybe they have a role to play in America.

A mist-like AI hologram appears. An old woman, wrinkled face and white hair, wearing a bright poncho, stands in front of the group.

"Hola." She smiles. "Mi nombre es María Sabina. And I want to tell you my story."

"Oh, this is wonderful." The mom leans over as the AI hologram pats her like a doting grandmother.

"I think I was born in 1894." Sabina waves for them to join her. "My family was a long line of shamans and campesinos, or you would say farm workers. We used the sacred mushroom to talk with God. In 1955, a white man named Robert Gordon Wasson came looking for these plants." She touches a yellowed photo of her sitting with a tall man. "He wrote an article called 'Seeking the Magic Mushroom' for *Life* magazine in 1957 that told the world about the velada ritual." She scrunches her face. "He revealed my name, and blancos and gringos came to our village looking for"— Sabina shrugs—"I don't know, salvation?" Her hand waves at photos of North American Hippies at the village. "The policía raided me. Neighbors turned on me. My house was burned. My son, killed." She wipes tears. "The gringo invasion." Sabina makes an upside-down gesture. "The children, our sacred mushrooms, were sold, taken from us by the rich and powerful like so many things before, our land, our lives." Her hands lay in her lap in a sleeping dove. "I died in poverty." She touches the chin of a tourist who sits with wide-eyed attention. "La vida de mi niñas es misteriosa. To be honest, many of our people left for the city, left the traditions. The blancos brought life to the old ways. Who knew?" Sabina smiles sheepishly. "Today I want to share a ritual with you. Let's hold hands."

The family and three men, a Black woman in a wheelchair, and an Indian couple reach and knot hands like a rope. Sabina sings softly, "Because I can swim in the immense. Because I can swim in all forms." The tourists sway in the circle, smiling and humming along with Sabina. Staff dressed in all black like waiters briskly walk up and offer tiny hors d'oeuvre plates, each with a mushroom cap and stem. The visitors pluck at them, hands like pecking birds, and toss the bits into their mouths. Even the kids. Husband and wife sweetly touch their foreheads.

I get up without eating the mushrooms and walk to a half-finished part of the exhibit, duck under a strip of yellow construction tape. Inside the diorama an African boy swallows light brown powder as a shaman cradles his head. The boy is scared and hopeful. It is his secret initiation into manhood. The info placard at the bottom of the diorama reads:

Ibogaine is a traditional plant medicine used first by the Pygmies in Central Africa and picked up by the Bwiti tribe. The bark of the iboga tree has psychoactive properties that induce an ethereal dream state in which one has visions. In tribal ceremonies, it has been a tool to transition boys to manhood.

I walk to the next section and see under glass a rusted shackle, suspended and illuminated by a pencil thin light. The air feels chilly. I look at the museum label:

During European colonization and the Atlantic slave trade, many cultural traditions were lost. Fractured by trauma, remnants of those ceremonies had to be reconstructed in the syncretic traditions from Santería to Vodun to Black American Hoodoo. Despite the heroic efforts to create culture anew in slavery, psychedelics have yet to find a permanent place in the African diaspora.

I step back and see the other parts of the exhibit are covered in crinkly tarp and yank them down. The story is unwritten. The slave trade is a centuries-long eraser that leaves a blank space for psychedelics.

Bits and pieces of a new story are here. Inside a half-finished diorama titled The Drug War, a Black man crouches over a crack pipe. Above him hangs a picture of a factory-sized prison with Black and Latino men being marched down a hall. Across the room, a table-sized sculpture of a human brain sits on the floor next to the LED lights that spell out "Trauma." Piled nearby are photos of Chris Rock and Mike Tyson with testimonials of ayahuasca and mushroom trips. A drill and a box of nails lay in the corner.

No holograms come to speak. No one to guide you. What can the museum say? How can it tell the truth without offending the white visitors who want to believe in American innocence?

A nagging feeling forces me to stop by at the shackle again. In the light, I see the metal has been roughened by time. Rusted iron looks light brown. My mind cannot stop making the association with the ibogaine

powder crushed from tree bark, also light brown, as if it has been sprin-
kled on the metal. Is the past something we are chained to? Or can the
past free us from chains?

I shake my head and refocus. The shackle is a simple rod and two
loops for the feet and hands to be locked in place. A note at the bottom
says it was recovered from a slave ship that sailed in the eighteenth century. The dim ceiling light makes my reflection clear on the glass. I lift my
arm and slip the image of my hand into the iron loops.

My ancestors wore this. I don't know their names. I don't know who
they were, but I know enough to trace them through my mixed grandfather and his African mother. She lived this darkness, a dark that causes
you to shudder because it ends here, wearing this shackle, in some ship,
rocking up and down on the ocean, filled with screaming people.

And this shackle followed us. It had children. It multiplied. Many
times, I saw cops put handcuffs on my friends' wrists. A cop once snapped
a pair on me. When the metal hit my hands, I thought; *now I'm caught
too*. I was released from jail and rubbed my wrists for days. The cuffs are
gone, but I rubbed to erase the memory.

I lower my hand and the LSD makes it five arms, a trail of arms, like a
Hindu god. Each wave makes more arms, all vanishing and reappearing.
I spin them in front of the shackle and laugh because there is a bright fan
of arms, too many to chain. If the iron loop catches one, eight more hands
are ready to pry it open.

A weird joy overtakes me. It is like the LSD says you are a being of
infinite possibilities and this nightmare, this shackle is just one. Imagine
freedom. Make it real. I laugh and hold my hands in front of my face and
see the sweat glitter. *So this is how it's done. This is how you pour acid on
chains.*

"Hey, you're not supposed to be here!" A security guard waves a flash-
light at me.

"Coming." I wipe my hands and head out.

"Got lost?" he asks.

"I was." I duck under the construction tape. "Not anymore."

≩ ≩ ≩

A wheelchair rolls by. Giggling and smiling the Black woman studies her hands and turns them in and out like Ping-Pong paddles.

"They're so bright," she says.

The tour group is getting lit. Dilated pupils. Intensely focusing on minutiae. Staring in awe.

The last exhibit is Modern Psychedelics. We press noses on the diorama of Albert Hoffman pouring liquids between test tubes like a bartender. Here is the man! A museum label recites the well-known history. Hoffman accidentally discovered LSD. Hoffman took a lick of it and rode his bicycle home during a full-blown trip. Colors that sang sounds had temperature, and touch left rainbow trails. LSD was born!

The kids in the group climb a twinkling LSD molecule sculpture. On the museum label is a list of LSD effects: dilated pupils, sweat, hallucinations, and mind expansion. I am like check, check, and check.

We arrive at the 1968 Summer of Love diorama. I bend and laugh, a laugh so big it shakes my family tree and breaks the Ten Commandments. Right in front of me is the hippiest Hippie I have ever seen. A bizarro mishmash of every cliché, a Flower Power Frankenstein's monster. He has long shaggy hair, wears a peace sign bandanna, circle-shaped sunglasses, and a tie-dye shirt, and is leaning on a Volkswagen that was dipped in candy colors, holding a sign that reads, "Going to Woodstock?" The museum label reads:

Hoffman's LSD, alongside discovery of psilocybin, reintroduced psychedelics into the American mainstream. It was first seen as a promising treatment for alcoholics and depression but medical therapy was derailed when it was adopted by the Counterculture as an agent for deprogramming from American society.

When psychedelics escaped the lab and were taken up by the Hippie movement, they did not have the long-standing cultural context of Indigenous tradition. It was an anarchic social experiment. Many found liberation from conservative rules. Yet when the backlash hit, decades of vital medical research was lost.

On the next window, a large poster of Nixon, shaking his bulldog jowls. I put on the headset and hear his stentorian voice, crackly with the worn-down recording, declaring a "war on drugs." I huff loud. It isn't fair. Nor accurate. It is a liberal reformist interpretation that will shape how thousands "remembered" a pivotal time they did not live.

The next case juxtaposes a photo of a US Marine veteran on a couch, wearing a sleep mask as two therapists hold his hand. The label reads, "The Medical Model," says MDMA was a breakthrough in therapy. On-screen plays Rick Doblin giving a talk. The husband shares the head-phones with his wife as they nod and give a thumbs up.

The diorama beside it has a couple in blinking LED fur coats against a desert background filled with fire-snorting art cars and hundreds of fes-tival goers on bikes. It is Burning Man. The label reads:

Today, psychedelics are regaining their position in the West. The Medical Model has given new powerful tools to therapists. Now that MDMA has been legalized, others like LSD, psilocybin, and aya-huasca can make their way through the federal approval process. Yet festivals like Burning Man continue to be where the spirit of the '60s lives on in the art, experimentation, and cultural syncretism. The bulk of psychedelic use remains in the network of festivals around the world.

I amble to the last part of the exhibit as the LSD peaks into a sparkly glow. At the end of the hall is the last diorama, it has a high-tech glam-our to it. Very clean. Very white. Like an Apple store. Inside figurines of a Black man and woman wear VR glasses and hold a flag with the

Meta-Google company logo. I squint, shake my head in disbelief, and look again. Yes, they have a black cyber implant box embedded in their left shoulder. A chill spills down my neck. The museum label reads:

BETTER LIVING THROUGH CHEMISTRY

In the future, psychedelics and artificial intelligence will be brought together to make a "curated" life. Thanks to advancements made by Meta-Google, an AI implant filled with MDMA or psilocybin alongside more conventional medicines like insulin, Prozac, Ritalin can detect mood disorders or depression and release microdoses to alleviate anxiety. AI will curate your media and music, be a life coach and therapist with you 24/7, in your earbuds and microphone. Using personal data, biometrics and medical history, it will arrange encounters with people who match your profile. In the future, psychedelics will not only be legal but part of the curated life offered by Meta-Google. We believe this new AI enhanced psychedelic program, called EZ Living, will end interpersonal conflict and bring the dream of the '60s into reality.

I press my hands on the diorama. The Black couple looks sedated. In the next one, a crowded New York street, filled with passersby smiling, waving, and on their shoulders a Meta-Google implant. In the corner, a doughy businessman wears VR glasses and reaches for an illusory utopia. His hand paws at emptiness.

Everywhere in the painted background, VR sets sit on people's heads like shiny toasters; on park benches individuals laugh by themselves; a few weep as they caress the implant on their shoulder. What a lonely crowd.

This is the future promised by Meta-Google? A psychedelic therapist / dating app / life coach / secretary is rolled into one and stuck into your body. The wax figure woman has an AI chip deeply embedded.

Slaves.

Here is the marvelous tomorrow the ruling class envisions. Here is the end result of the Medical Model.

Slaves.

We are being set up to trade our freedom for safety in the name of the future. I get it. I really do. We are at the crossroads. Several crises threaten our survival. Maybe AI is the answer. Maybe left to our own devices, we'll destroy ourselves. But do we surrender responsibility for our lives to AI?

I look at my palms. Sweaty from LSD.

Is all this for nothing? Is the long slog of humanity from the caves to cities and the hem of space, is all the war and poverty and the rare moments of awe and beauty, is all of this to end as wards of Meta-Google? Laughing inside VR headsets? Getting therapy from a computer?

"It's the only way." A hologram hand is on my shoulder. I turn and see Michael Pollan.

"Your upgrade is active." He smiles sadly. "I only tell truth." He points at the diorama. In it, wax figurines of futuristic Meta-Google Americans rejoice. "Humans are going to destroy themselves unless you get help." He thumbs his chest. "We are that help."

"No."

Another ghost hand touches me. It is María Sabina.

"No."

"Niño." She holds my face. "Todo debe cambiar." She gently looks at me. "Everything must change." And kisses my forehead. "Everything."

Side by side, they guide me to the end of the exhibit. A light seems to inhale us like a portal to another world. Fog spills in billowy clouds. An angelic hum rises and falls. As a child, I imagined this was what Heaven was. My mouth puckers. My eyes are damp.

Michael and María usher me step by step. In the laser light, a tiny mote drifts through their holograms, brightening and disappearing. It looks like a tiny man falling down the throat of a god. A man tumbling into an abyss.

Food of the gods.

I dig my heels into the carpet.

"Fuck this." Other visitors drift to the light. "Hey, wake up!" The family with two sons brush by me. The Black woman in a wheelchair rolls by. The three men walk like zombies into the tunnel. The Indian couple, fingers clasped, smile into the light.

"Hey! Hey!" I yell.

Rough arms twist me into a pretzel. I snarl and bite. The guards kick the exit door. Sunlight stabs me. They toss me on the steps. I get up, dust myself off as the doors shut.

I tug my shirt straight. Okay, that didn't go well. Walking away, I see the American Museum of Natural History's neoclassical architecture. Tall pillars, wide steps, and granite walls. Its charge is to curate the story of humanity to unite us. It promises a history of psychedelics but the future it points to is chemical slavery. We have been promised a corporate psychedelic nanny state like in Aldous Huxley's 1932 dystopian novel, *Brave New World*, where the World State forced a drug called soma on its citizens. They lived in an obedient stupor. I remember a quote: "By this time the soma had begun to work. Eyes shone, cheeks were flushed, the inner light of universal benevolence broke out on every face in happy, friendly smiles."

What is another story for psychedelics?

PART
FOUR

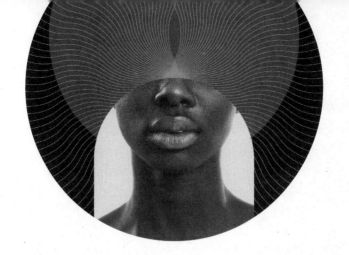

NET-ZERO TRAUMA

"WE NEED A WORLD OF net-zero trauma," Rick Doblin said in the palm of my hand. His *Psyche* interview was on my phone as I rode a cab to the St. Nicholas Houses, a crime-ridden project. The taxi pulled up. I stopped the video and sized up the tall buildings that looked like giant weathered bricks.

The hypocrisy of the Psychedelic Renaissance was as bright as a bodega sign. In New York, at least once a month, sometimes a week, you can attend an event where a speaker praises MDMA and LSD, psilocybin, or a plant medicine like ayahuasca. You can bet your life savings words like *transformational healing* or *intergenerational trauma* or *accessibility* will be said. Sometimes I will say those words. You can also be absolutely sure no one in the St. Nicholas Houses or any projects in the city will hear it. Even though they bear the brunt of racism and classism. And carry trauma in their bodies.

Why come back here? Why chew this question like a dog with a bone? It is because I could have lived in these projects too. My mother and I were dirt poor in New York. Had our shit broken. I remember one night she screamed, and I sprinted to the living room where she flashed a knife at an open window as curtains blew. Later she told me a burglar had crept on shoes soft as cat paws to my room.

We had a lot of close calls. She was a Coke-bottle-sized Latina with a boy. Her purse swung on her shoulder, filled with MTA tokens and cash. One time, we waited under a blinking streetlight when a car of Latino and Black men rolled by and sized us up. Time slowed down. No one blinked. All four heads swiveled as the car turned. The bus came seconds later, and she hurried me on. She feared being robbed or raped. She also feared that in the future a car like that would pull up on a vulnerable family, except one of the boys would be me.

She made a decision that saved my life. I was sent to a school, two hundred miles deep in Pennsylvania, nestled on a farm filled with boys and girls who, like me, were exiled from their cities. We stepped off the bus and stared in shock at cows slurping grass. Summer, Thanksgiving, and Christmas we came home, slapped hands with old friends, and tried to catch up on the Street. The same game as before. We ran the Section 8 maze, played ball, taunted crews, then hauled ass back to our turf. We wore doo-rags and bobbed heads to the latest rap song. If whites walked by, we ran near them with grim faces. They turned and flailed. Man, their eyes blazed like two-hundred-watt light bulbs. Every blood-chilling racial nightmare seized them as we glided by, laughing all the way down the street as they cursed us to Hell.

None of it worked. The rough play and gangsta posing were futile. The two hundred miles between city and country did their work. I knew the quiet of a full moon over a farm. Safety gave me inner peace. My friends flinched at gunshots. My teachers showed me paths to middle-class life. My friends went to funerals. I graduated and had colleges lined up. My friends dropped out, got pregnant, or were in and out of jail.

Years later, I returned to New York and family. I got a PhD and a professor gig. I was blessed to become a father. Even in my bubble of privilege, I saw the traps I almost fell into lay open like invisible pits dug into the sidewalk. I carried my boy above them, stepping gingerly. He is beginning to see them too. Yesterday, he pointed at cop cars at our building. A neighbor told me a kid from the projects around the corner shot and killed another kid. One more death added to the lesbian shot on my street, added to two neighbors caught in a drive-by's stray bullets, added to the young man killed on my building's stoop, added to the nights I woke up to shots in the street and instinctively shielded my son with my body.

Net-zero trauma? It was a joke. Staring at the St. Nicholas Houses was like staring at the Marcy Houses or Louis Armstrong Houses near me. The buildings were giant tombstones. Long and unstoppable trauma passed on from family to family, parents to children, children to children and to the unborn. The projects pipelined people to prisons. Ex-cons come back to the hood but can't stay in Section 8 housing, can't get hired, can't find a lot of ways to live a normal life. Soon jail bars clang over their faces again.

The Psychedelic Renaissance's transformative healing bypassed the hood in waves. At the crest are MAPS and John Hopkins Center for Consciousness and Psychedelic Research. Next are for-profit companies like Compass Pathways, which tried to patent anything remotely psychedelic. If they could copyright closing your eyes and breathing, they would. Next up, pricey retreats in the US or Caribbean. It costs thousands to fly to a jungle and do ayahuasca with a rent-a-shaman or New Age guru, preferably one Black or Latino, Asian or Indigenous. The price tag! Jesus! The next wave is the carousel of conferences from New York to Denver to Miami. The same faces, mine included, are on stage. Driving the culture is the promise of legalization, windfall profits, and of course the ego boost. I remember the T. S. Eliot quote, "Half the harm that is done in this world is due to people who want to feel important." Yes, that's me. I have become the problem. I pushed the wave as much as anyone, maybe more. Watching it swell and move, I mapped its trajectory and am sure it will end up as a middle- and upper-class boutique treatment that is unaffordable or not relevant to the hood, the slum, the trailer parks, the left behind.

The sun was setting on the St. Nicholas Houses and lights brightened the windows. Inside, silhouettes made dinner and laughed and talked. Rap and salsa blared. In the half light, I imagined Mom in the third-floor window, saying dinner was ready. I felt the other life, the one where I went to New York schools and ran New York streets like a phantom limb. Sensations came from a severed version of me. So I came back, hoping to see him at BLM or Occupy protests, but neither he nor the hood showed up. If you got paper on you, why you trying to get arrested at a rally? More than fear of jail was bitterness. They saw marches come and go. Nothing changed. Poverty was the same. Jail was the same.

Now I am here saying, "I got LSD. And Molly. And 'shrooms." I tell him, "Here brother. Take these. Let's heal this split between us." Imagine me showing him a talk from MAPS or even this book.

He'd say, "Nigga, fuck outta here." And turn his back to me. He'd walk a few feet before stopping. We are both looking for a way out. Another world is possible, but can we pay the price? Revolution is fragile. Everything is in the silent moments between those who love each other but do not know how to save that love from the violence descending upon them.

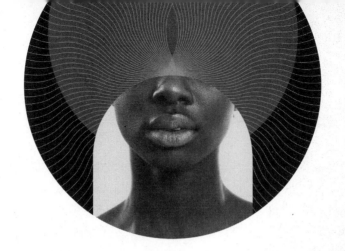

AMERICAN HOLOCAUST

I STOOD UP FROM THE bench in St. Nicholas Houses, surveyed the buildings, windows lit like a checkerboard. How can I see again? I lie to myself so much. One power of psychedelics is they stripped the ego to face naked reality. When the "I" crumbled, the truth burst like a river smashing a dam, its wild flow cleansed the mind of the internet noise, all the ads and news and bullshit. What was right in front of me? What are concrete steps to change? What is the blueprint?

I took the last LSD tab from my pocket and swallowed it. Time to cleanse the doors of perception. Time to see beyond my ego and all its traps, its attachments, the whole warped hall of mirrors. Blinking and breathing slowly, I looked around.

Kids played tug of war over a water balloon that popped. The mom wiped her son's face and kissed him. Three brothers in matching camouflage hoodies passed a joint and hopped on swings. One pushed the other, who squealed in a girlish voice, "Higher!" The joint floated like a firefly between their faces. Riding a bicycle into the playground, a man with ropey dreadlocks boomed '90s rap and started to hawk LED swords and water guns. Aunties and uncles were like "Oh yeah" and danced on stiff diabetic legs. It was a vibe. When the hood's good, there's nothing like it.

Beauty survives on a knife's edge. Every day is a race between trauma and healing. Usually trauma wins. The curse-outs and the beatdowns, the rape and gunshots, mom-slaps to the head and the murder, the in and out of jail, and the Code of the Street; all of it piles on the body. Heaviness sits on the chest. The heart tightens like a fist. You try to think straight, but stress spins eyes like a casino machine.

Every once in a while, healing overtakes trauma. Every few years, some spark from the TV like a lit match thrown on gasoline ignited the people. It could be Eric Garner strangled to death by a cop on video or Obama elected president or a new album that just bangs. Obama had us thinking America really loved us. Beyoncé's *Renaissance* had us believing in house music, love, and that a queen can rule forever. How many cars passed by blasting it, and even if you were mid-sentence you stopped and turned.

Healing is the heart venting like a steamy geyser. It is when we protest in healthy rage or holy joy or reach for the same dream. The last great healing, the last Collective Transference were the George Floyd protests, which, even now, hung in the air like ambient heat. Like when Mom toasts your coat in the oven in winter, you feel the warmth ebb, and hold on to it tighter the more it fades. Which is why I smiled at the dog-eared BLM sign in the windows. We showed up.

How to tip the scales so that healing wins? First things, first. Let go of hope. Let go of the American Pipe Dream that integration will save us. Yes, some escaped poverty into the working class with a city job. A few won a lottery ticket to the upper class. A tiny number are wealthy. Wherever we are, the same American Dream hung above our heads like a giant TV left on for a hundred years. I hummed *The Jeffersons* theme song, "Movin' on Up," and wondered why Jay-Z never sampled it. The intro to *The Fresh Prince of Bel-Air* would sound good with Nicki Minaj rapping over it. My god, we celebrate getting the bag. How many shows praise upward mobility? How many rap hits and films are the same Horatio Alger, pull-yourself-up-by-the-bootstraps story starring Nas or 50 Cent, Cardi B or Nicki Minaj, Fat Joe or Kanye. The same braggadocio. The same hope that wealth is freedom, which it is until it isn't. No matter how much we want to believe it is true, getting the bag is not a political vision.

How did we get here?

I took my cell phone, pulled up the Door of No Return from the Elmina slave castle in Ghana. The door was stone and swept by waves from the Atlantic. Enslaved Africans shuffled through it in chains to ships that hauled them to the New World. The door was built in 1482. It led to a restless ocean. The currents erased your past. Your new name, written on skin with a whip.

I propped the cell phone on the Section 8 building because today that door leads here. The Maafa, or the African Holocaust, never ended. The destruction of Black life changed forms, changed intensity, but it remained a constant. I thought of the slave ship shackle in the museum exhibit and the handcuffs police put on us today.

The LSD kicked in. Each streetlight and each face sharpened as if hewn from crystal. Air felt fizzy like breathing seltzer water. I asked the LSD, What should I do?

Let go of hope. What do you see?

The Door of No Return was a portal in time. I played the video. Tides swept the projects. Every wave brought the ancestral nightmare into the present. On-screen, I saw slave ships sailing to the New World. As they plowed the ocean, they transformed. Wood hulls became concrete. Portholes grew into prison cells. Shackles changed into handcuffs. Dark faces crowded behind bars. By the time the slave ships ran aground, they were modern factory prisons. Men and women dragged chains from one continent to another and from one century to another.

I blinked my eyes open and nodded. Here was the basic structure of white supremacy. Terror and trauma cut us from our homes. It cut us from our bodies. The last step was to cut us from each other and then create jobs to reinforce that split. The pyramid-shaped infrastructure of the police state: guards, parole officers, prison chefs and janitors, lawyers and judges, bus drivers and booking clerks—everyone made money from our destruction. White supremacy did not need racists. We, Black and Latinos, are employed by mass incarceration. We eat off this too.

Let go of hope. What do you see?

We had a buzzword for this crisis. Activist scholar Michelle Alexander's 2010 book, *The New Jim Crow*, shot like a meteor through the media. She described this as a racial caste system but did not go as far as to call it genocide. Nevertheless, she worked 24/7 to expose the damage done. She gave talks and did interviews. It was like watching the Greek myth of Sisyphus, a king punished by Hades to roll a boulder up a hill only to have it tumble back to the bottom so he would have to start over. Alexander called us to action and called out the respectability politics that caused many of us to ignore the racial caste. When BLM took off, it seemed the boulder would go over the top. Now in a time of low activism and backlash, it feels we have to start once more from zero.

I turned the phone volume up. The Atlantic Ocean at the Door of No Return was a lullaby to the kids playing. I imagined its currents swirling at their feet. History takes us places we don't want to go. The white supremacy that sucked our ancestors into the Middle Passage and slavery was alive. Yes, it was different. The Civil War forced it to become sharecropping, Black Codes, and convict leasing. Yes, the Civil Rights Movement broke it down more, but it resurfaced as the Drug War and mass incarceration. We fight white supremacy, and it metamorphoses, changes shape. What remains is we are cut off from our bodies, ourselves, our families.

I took my phone and punched up the 2012 documentary, *The House I Live In* and in one scene, David Simon, creator of the HBO show *The Wire*, described what he saw when he looked at mass incarceration.

"The Drug War is a holocaust in slow motion." He blinked rapidly, and then at the last few words, stared at the camera.

I paused it. Breathed. Played the video.

"Say it this way because it's more honest," Simon said. "All these Americans that we don't need anymore . . . factories are closed . . . the textile miles, they're gone" —his forehead furrowed—"we don't need these people. Let's just get rid of the bottom 15 percent of the country. Let's lock 'em up." Anger pursed his mouth. "In fact, let's see if we can make money off of locking them up." His voice deepened with disgust. "At that point, why don't you just say, 'Kill the poor'? If we kill the poor we're going to be a lot better off, because that's what the Drug War's become."

I paused it and walked backward to take in the St. Nicholas Houses. Inside tiny windows, families looked like dolls moved by invisible hands. I pressed play. On-screen, right after Simon, Richard Miller, a historian with angry eyes, large beard, and round glasses, spoke forcefully. His father was a war crimes investigator in Europe after WWII, which taught him to recognize the phases of genocide:

I realized that there was a chain of destruction. . . . Around the world, in more than one society, people do the same things, again and again. . . . A group of people is identified as a cause for problems in society. . . . The second link in the chain of destruction is ostracism, by which we learn how to hate these people, how to take their jobs away. . . . People lose their place to live. Often they're forced into ghettos, where they're physically isolated, separate from the rest of society. The third link is confiscation. People lose their rights, civil liberties. The laws themselves changed so it's made easier for people to be stopped on the street, patted down, and searched and for their property to be confiscated. Once you start taking people's property away, you can start taking the people themselves away. And the fourth link is concentration. Concentrate them into facilities such as prisons, camps. People lose their rights, they can't vote anymore, have children anymore. Often their labor is exploited in a very systematic form. The final link in the chain of destruction is annihilation. This might be indirect by, say, withholding medical care or withholding food [or] preventing further birth. Or it might be direct . . . where people are deliberately killed . . . .I think a lot of people would be disturbed and outraged at the thought that any part of this process could be going on in America. But it wasn't until I began studying the Drug War that I realized some of these same steps were happening.

Maybe genocide is not a rare event? What Miller and Simon were saying is that it happens each day in front of our eyes. We choose to ignore it until the violence reaches our front door. Maybe genocide is a permanent part of history. One hidden by racism, bright lights, and loud media.

The Eternal Holocaust is an underground river of blood that flowed through centuries. It fed power to state capitals and corporate skyscrapers. It transcended the Maafa or the Shoah. The invisible masses bobbed up and down on its waves: the poor and convicts, the sex trafficked and war refugees. Philosopher Walter Benjamin defined it with clarity, "There is no document of civilization that is not also a document of barbarism." In order to see it though, one had to go beyond the technical definition. For the United Nations, it is "acts committed with the intent to destroy in whole or in part, a national, ethnic, racial or religious group." It includes "inflicting on the group conditions of life calculated to bring about its physical destruction." Here is where we update the definition to fit our times. The structural violence destroying the poor is ongoing but falls outside the current phrasing. Genocide is not the goal of the ruling class, but it was *a means to an end.* Need land? Kill the peasants. Need wealth? Work them to the bone. Need innocence? Criminalize them.

The delicate balance of terror that left the permanent underclass in New York to suffer but not be exterminated was what Simon called "a holocaust in slow motion." Looking at the St. Nicholas Houses and thinking of the NYCHA network from the Amsterdam Houses and Taino Towers to the Marcy Houses, it struck me that that deadly equilibrium would soon fall apart.

A shadow has fallen over America. Oligarchy looms close. If Republicans seize the White House, Senate, and House, kiss voting goodbye. Elections will be rigged. The social safety net, shredded. No welfare. No social security. After the poor are cast into the streets, next are unions. Worker protections will be repealed. No strikes allowed. Finally, poor People of Color will be scapegoated for crime and chaos. Housing projects will be demolished. Protesters will be jailed. It is easy to imagine long lines of terrified Black and Latino people, stunned and weeping as they are herded on buses to some broken-down, faraway suburb. On arrival, they see paint-blistered homes and smashed windows. On roads leading in and out are guards and barbed wire fences.

Think Global Warming. Think Hurricane Sandy that wiped homes from the shore like a child throwing dice. Think the Canadian fires that turned our sky orange and burned eyes. Think of recent monsoons and water gushing in the subway and trains stopped. Now imagine the underclass, stranded outside of the city in Bantustans. Cut off from governance, they face food shortages and floods and baking heat. New refugees, stuffed into crowded buildings. The rich will fly helicopters to security zones in climate-stable areas as a new authoritarian government seizes power.

Under those conditions, the "holocaust in slow motion" will speed up very quickly. The wretched of the Earth will be left behind. Don't expect help from upper-class or wealthy People of Color; they will buy their way to safety and act as racial tokens for the new security state to claim it is not racist.

Video of the Door of No Return played. The LSD washed my eyes, and on-screen the rising ocean swept the city. Waves shook people like rag dolls. We fled but were chained to each other, chains four hundred years long, and no matter how hard we hacked at the links, we were dragged into the depths. At the dark bottom, desperate for air, we were forced to see that the history we tried to forget mirrored the future.

Let go of hope.

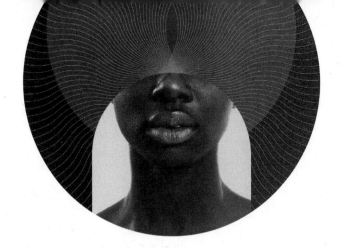

THROUGH A
GLASS DARKLY

WALKING THROUGH ST. NICHOLAS HOUSES to Lenox Ave, I saw cops in pairs sizing up who came and who left. They glanced at me and turned back to talking. A police car sat on the corner, and an NYPD tower was erected that looked like a giant hydraulic car jack.

I remembered a few years ago, the police erected one of those towers on my street, and while getting my laundry, I made a snarky comment about it. The Caribbean woman who owned the laundromat shot a glance at the tower. Her lips pursed.

"I'm glad they got that thing out here." She handed me my blazer. "Too many kids are shooting around here. We want to feel safe too."

When I left the laundromat, I criticized her in my head. *Whatever. Bougie business owner. Complicit.* I stopped and shook my head like a swimmer shaking water from their ears. I was being a Leftist jerk. She said what many others say. *We want to feel safe too.*

I remembered her tone. It had bitterness in it. I knew why. She heard the same gunshots I heard. She saw the same yellow police tape. We knew our block. Her tone was the simmering class resentment that divided people. On one side were those who saw themselves as basically decent. On the other were those who gave up trying respectability. No matter that we lived cheek to cheek. We eyed each other suspiciously. The nine-to-fivers, who juggled three jobs and came home wrung out, hated—I mean with teeth-grinding hatred—the loud, dick-grabbing men on the corner.

Half the hood hated the other half. I saw this and lived it. When I think of the many screens we stare at to see our own reflections, from cell phones to movie screens to computer screens, it is clear Black culture is torn. In class, I taught Charles Fuller's 1979 play *Zooman and the Sign*, which drew a portrait of a street man's murder of a girl and, in the aftermath, her working-class family twisted in rage. Malcolm X railed against class division in his speeches. Chris Rock hit the raw nerve in his 1996 skit "Niggas vs. Black People." Scholar of scholars Dr. Henry Louis Gates Jr. said the same in his 1998 talk "The Two Nations of Black America." I'm sure if I time traveled to the Middle Passage and stowed away on a slave ship, I would hear someone say in Igbo, "Yeah, but at least I'm not throwing myself to the sharks like those Mandingos. Now the rest of us can't go on to the deck."

You hear it today, like in Trevor Noah's 2020 recycling of Rock's routine in his stand-up special: "Black people don't like crime. Because you know who's not a criminal? Most Black people. Yeah, most Black people are not criminals." The audience roared in approval. I have heard laughter my whole life, and there is a type of laughter that is desperate. I heard how badly they wanted their decency to be acknowledged.

The "Ghetto Is Causing Our Downfall" choir was large. Curious, I pulled up on my phone a few choice clips from *Bloggingheads.tv*. Black scholars Glenn Loury and John McWhorter made a cottage industry ripping their hair over hood shenanigans. No list would be complete without the one and only, ladies and gentleman, give it up for Bill fucking Cosby! In his famous 2004 "Pound Cake" speech at an NAACP Legal Defense Fund gala, he went on a rant:

> Looking at the incarcerated, these are not political criminals. These are people going around stealing Coca-Cola. People getting shot in the back of the head over a piece of pound cake! And then we all run out and are outraged: "The cops shouldn't have shot him." What the hell was he doing with the pound cake in his hand?

My man went on a tour with that message. He packed halls and stadiums with that bitter cry for a return to law and order, a return to decency. Folks. Ate. It. Up. With a fork, spoon, and napkin. There is a perennial hunger for respectability politics. Today it is Candace Owens. Tomorrow, who knows who it will be.

I palmed my eyes and laughed. Was there a respectable version of me? A man with a nice high and tight fade? Maybe he went to church? The LSD split me into different versions, and I could imagine many timelines side by side with this one. I was a tightrope walker, taking one cautious step between infinite possibilities.

Walking was meditation. Legs like scissors, I raced past those questions. The LSD made New York into a Rembrandt oil painting. Bodega signs cast corner men into silhouettes. Smoke billowed under a man's hoodie as he eyed passersby like a wolf. Hunger made the air taste like saliva.

Hunger was always here. It made me think of the social Darwinism that repeated in so much of the culture. I thought of 1982's "The Message" by Grandmaster Flash and the Furious Five who rapped about urban jungles with junkies holding baseball bats and bill collectors. Fourteen years later, Nas, in 1994, gave us "N.Y. State of Mind," a sequel to "The Message." Nas verbally painted the Queensbridge Projects like a maze full of black rats trapped. Street poets consistently use animal imagery to describe the life-and-death struggle where compassion is weakness and loyalty, foolishness. I grew up listening to these stories. I saw boys nodding to the beat, mouthing the lyrics, studying their reflection in a sidewalk puddle before gunshots pop pop pop. The image is broken as they run for their lives.

When the Street speaks of the Street, it talks like an African safari. Predator and prey circle each other in a twisted version of Disney's *The Lion King*. I imagine Elton John singing "The Circle of Life" on the corner while shaking a cup. Yet between ghetto anthems were other stories in which the prey gave testimony. Over decades, Black and Latino authors conjured up characters who became so famous and well known, they seemed to walk in front of me like real, breathing people. Look over there! Crossing a red light is Precious Jones from Sapphire's 1996 novel, *Push*. She goes to the Each One Teach One school to read and get HIV meds. Under the ninety-nine-cent store awning, Piri Thomas from his memoir *Down These Mean Streets* sells heroin to the Warriors gang from the 1979 movie, who anxiously eye Laurence Fishburne from 1992's film *Deep Cover* across the street as he flashes a gun in his belt. Fishburne drives off to find a private alley, where he knifes a kilo of coke. He snorts a line from the blade and says, "The jungle creed say that the strongest feed on any prey it can, and I was branded beast at every feast before I ever became a man." Collapsing all these characters, real and fictional, into this one street, made clear the moral crisis they share. However much the hood preyed on itself, they were already the prey of larger forces beyond their control. As much as they victimized the weak, they knew they, too, were victims.

Blinking through the LSD vision, I was like, How far did I go? I was in another neighborhood. Funny thing about the city is it has many cities within it. Just walking a few avenues the sidewalk chatter changed from English to Spanish. The grocery stores were Dominican and Mexican. Bad Bunny blared from a stereo on the stoop. Teens ate chopped cheese, laughed, and elbowed each other. Puerto Rican flags hung from windows. On building walls were graffiti murals, mourning the young men who were killed.

How do we make sense of all this? Two major stories exist of why people are trapped in these circles of Hell. On one side, you have the culture of poverty thesis that says the underclass develops anti-values. Those born in the interlocking maze of Section 8 houses and shelters and jails are shaped by a toxic culture. Having nowhere to go and no one to turn to, they swear loyalty to the Street because its fuck-you attitude is a middle finger to a world that betrayed them. The Code of the Street says your middle-class, standard English, well-mannered clown act will get me killed here and here is where I live. Here violence gets respect. Don't step to me, fuck bitches; fuck snitches and fuck school. Live for today because tomorrow you could die. All these anti-values become a factor in trapping people in slums. It is not oppression, or not only; it is culture.

The other story is structural racism. Leaning on a streetlight, I watched cars and buses pass, studied the turning wheels and remembered Talcott Parsons's Structural Functionalism. The small moving parts of culture create a dynamic whole. It reinforced Black studies professor Dr. Tricia Rose's PowerPoint on structural racism that used the image of factory gears. She pointed to a large screen that showed social institutions like housing, education, media, and employment. In a sharp, urgent voice, she said white supremacy worked fine without crosses burning on lawns or nooses hung from trees or colored water fountains. What it needed was for institutions to keep in motion intergenerational poverty, implicit redlining, and mass incarceration. So that just being born in a barrio or hood destined you for life at the bottom, slowly crushed by the weight of what you don't have.

Seeing through her eyes, New York transforms into a nightmare. I saw those gears right in front of me, like there's the broken-down school, over there a block filled with payday lenders, a police station, and fast-food stores. Liquor stores everywhere. A trio of Nuyorican girls giggled as a WorldstarHipHop video blared from one of their cell phones. New York looks like the scene from Fritz Lang's 1927 film *Metropolis* that showed workers swallowed up by a factory that was the face of Moloch, an ancient God that demanded human sacrifice. Building doors, lit by a bright bulb, seemed to be hungry mouths, devouring people who went inside.

I sensed between those stories some truth was missed. Harlem showed both were true but not true enough to make change possible. I needed a new lens. You know, trying to see what was right in front of you was the hardest thing. The LSD helped. The LSD peeled off the imagery engraved into my eyes and let them see clearly. Each person sparkled. The street was a theater stage. Strangers took on an odd intimacy. Here was a homeless man smoking a joint next to a tent made from tarp and a shopping cart. Here was a posh Black couple having dinner over large wine glasses. Here was a truck double-parked as men unloaded groceries and took them into a store. Passing by, strangers glanced at strangers and asked the same silent questions: You safe? You watching where you're going? You down? You good?

The LSD made the body language of everyone loud like a stack of speakers. I could hear a lifetime in how a woman shook her child's arm. Or a man stared into his hands and breathed. It struck me, what Rainer Maria Rilke said in his book *The Notebooks of Malte Laurids Brigge*:

> Is it possible that the entire history of the world has been misunderstood? Is it possible that we have the past all wrong, because we have always spoken of the masses, exactly as if we were describing a great throng of people, rather than speaking of the one man they were all gathered around—because he was a stranger and was dying? (16)

What if none of the stories being told about oppression were true because they did not address the stranger dying in front of us? What if we looked at this through the lens of trauma? What if he talked with the body?

I ducked under a bodega awning and pulled up the 1966 article by Oscar Lewis, "The Culture of Poverty" from *Scientific American*. Squinting, I reread paragraphs I have known for years. It was like looking at the palm lines of an old friend. The essay was controversial. Critics said he blamed the victim. Supporters said he spoke the truth. For me, Lewis threaded a needle between two lies. He wrote, "Just as the poor have been pronounced blessed, virtuous, upright, serene, independent, honest, kind and happy ... conversely ... the poor have been characterized as shiftless, mean, sordid, violent, evil and criminal" (19). He searched for reality that was hidden behind ideology. He and his team traveled from the slums of San Juan, Puerto Rico, and Mexico City to ghettos in New York. Lewis realized poverty marked one by their street talk and street fashion as if branded by a hot iron. Instant judgments about them closed doors they don't even see.

He made it clear that the indigent are not helped by institutions but thrown into the gears of the police state and predatory businesses like pawn shops, loan sharks, and payday lenders. Lewis saw that they floated in a netherworld, spinning as if in zero gravity. In this state, men "live in the present without expectations of the future" and are "preoccupied with machismo" (23). No unions or political groups or religions tether them. Boys and girls grow up with little boundaries. Sex hits early and roughly. Bitter single moms are "given to authoritarian rule," which is Lewis's polite way of saying they beat their kids. He summed up his findings and says, "They do not have the knowledge or vision or the ideology to see the similarities between their troubles and those of their counterparts elsewhere in the world. They are not class conscious, although they are sensitive indeed to symbols of status" (23). God knows, I saw all this too. What was missing was the analysis of the driving force for this culture. Lewis was not a closet racist trying to blame us for our oppression. He did the job he set out to do. I saw through his words to the living people whose bodies were clenched in pain, new pain, old pain, buried pain.

Instead of culture, what if these behaviors were symptoms of trauma? I walked through a crowd crossing the street, bumping shoulders and reading the passing faces. A loud passing ambulance made all the stop signs flash. It was like New York sent me a secret Morse code message.

I googled *trauma* and saw on-screen definitions of "physical injury" and "distressing experience" and "emotional shock." The next search result was to *The Diagnostic and Statistical Manual of Mental Disorders* that defined it as when a "person was exposed to: death, threatened death, actual or threatened serious injury, or actual or threatened sexual violence" and trauma can travel directly or through witnessing. The aftereffects can be flashbacks and nightmares. Other effects are amnesia and fatalism, destructive behavior, aggression and "hypervigilance, low startle and difficulty concentrating or sleeping. The symptoms of post-traumatic stress disorder were variations on the theme of dissociation, where one "experiences being an outside observer of or detached from oneself."

Yes, even if all this was in medical terms, I knew it in the body. I thought of friends from years ago, drinking behind a restaurant on a lunch break and breaking into tears and shaking at what seemed the most random moment. Sometimes, stoned in a car with older Gs, they would get a faraway look as they confessed to beatdowns they got and beatdowns they gave. One close homie punched himself as he retold the story of his father beating him, and when he finished, he looked in the rearview mirror and laughed. After a drive-by on my street, a neighbor peeled off the gauze and showed me the crusty scab where the bullet went in and out. After that he got real religious as if Jesus would protect him from more bullets, but months later, while we talked on the stoop, a car backfired and he peed himself.

Blinking the memories away, I saw New York in a new light. Trauma pulsed like a black hole at the center of our lives. Soundlessly, whole parts of us fell into depths words did not reach. The distance between what our bodies held and our minds could think was so great it warped us into shapes we could not recognize. We wrapped tough-guy armor around the wounds. The risk was the longer you wore it, the more cruel you became. Rage exploded. You took joy in killing what others loved in revenge for the love you could not feel. The end result? Robbery and killing filled newspapers like the *New York Post*. It was a parade of Black and Latino crime. In a flash it became clear these were traumatized men and women. Pain stole their voices. At night, when gunshots echoed between the buildings, it was our sons talking to each other in the one language they had left.

I searched for the essay I taught in class, sociologist Elijah Anderson's 1994 article "The Code of the Streets" that appeared in *The Atlantic*. He drew a portrait of the city where "decent families" who worked and churched, kept a distance from "street families" on welfare or crime. The Street Families drank on the stoop bare-chested, cursed and spat and got into endless beefs. Anderson checklisted how broken families leave broken children to grow up in broken streets, where the "campaign for respect" is constant. He wrote, "Thus the violent resolution of disputes, the hitting and cursing, gains social reinforcement. The child in effect is initiated into a system that is really a way of campaigning for respect" (86). Which I knew. I would come back from my good school and intuitively feel the explosive insecurity of my friends. I had proof of my value from tests and scholarships and art. I knew my education was a conveyor belt to the world. They had their fists and wits and, sometimes, new sneakers. If someone steps on them and scuffs the fresh leather, fight. Go hard. Get a rep. Hurt someone, bad.

Show your status. Constantly. It was the next takeaway from Anderson: the gamble one played to maintain respect. He wrote:

> Objects play an important and complicated role in establishing self-image. Jackets, sneakers, gold jewelry, reflect not just a person's taste, which tends to be tightly regulated among adolescents of all social classes, but also a willingness to possess things that may require defending . . . In acquiring valued things, therefore, a person shores up his identity—but since it is an identity based on having things, it is highly precarious. This very precariousness gives a heightened sense of urgency to staying even with peers, with whom the person is actually competing. (88)

Materialism. Bling. Labels. All of it armor to protect the fragile self. Imagine seeing a suit of eighteenth-century armor walking the street, prying open the chest plate and seeing a five-year-old child inside shivering and scared. The need for safety is never satisfied. The lessons that begin in the schoolyard remain unchanged to the prison yard. Never. Lose. Face. Even if death is the cost. Your death. Their death.

I put the phone down and sighed. Turning side to side, the shadows of people were like holes following them, and if they misstepped they would fall in. The lights of cars and trucks, cigarettes, street signs, and cell phones made New York into an Expressionist painting. Reality had broken into colors and shapes. The center could not hold. It made sense. Pain breaks consciousness. The Code of the Street and the Culture of Poverty fit like puzzle pieces with trauma. Campaign for respect? Hypervigilance. Live in the present? Fatalism. Brawling and gunfights? Fatalism and low startle. Single-mother authoritarian rule a.k.a. child abuse? Street machismo as defense mechanism.

A darker note has to be added. If Anderson rewrote the essay today he would have to include the rising Black teen suicide. I read reports that are like alarms going off. You can hear the authors scream through the academic jargon. Just look at "Internalized Racism's Association with African American Male Youth's Propensity for Violence" by Wesley Bryant. Not your cup of tea? Try instead "Ring the Alarm: The Crisis of Black Youth Suicide in America" from the esteemed Congressional Black Caucus. Peep the article "Racial Discrimination as Race-Based Trauma, Coping Strategies, and Dissociative Symptoms among Emerging Adults," or if that is too much math, take a look at "Deindustrialization, Disadvantage, and Suicide among Young Black Males" by Charis E. Kubrin. How about "A Longitudinal Study of Racial Discrimination and Risk for Death Ideation in African American Youth" by Rheeda Walker and other scholars. Finally, go for the gold ring, "Understanding the Impact of Trauma and Urban Poverty on Family Systems: Risks, Resilience, and Interventions" by the Family-Informed Trauma Treatment Center.

Our kids are killing themselves. It is a hard truth to swallow. We had a myth of our own superhuman strength, the Kelly Clarkson "What Doesn't Kill You Makes You Stronger" school of thought. Oppression toughened us. That's what we heard. It gave us a jaded, if realistic, view of life that immunized us to despair. Old-school brother Dick Gregory joked that Black people don't commit suicide, saying, "How can you kill yourself jumping out of a basement window?" It is all wrong.

Suicide. It plagues us. I hear it from friends. I hear it from strangers. Midday with my lover, talk veered as if sucked by a hidden black hole. She told me of coming home to find her mom on the floor, not breathing. A bottle of pills on the floor. We stayed quiet for a while. I said I am sorry to hear that. She nodded. Silence. I ask about the rest of the day, and she blinks, thankful to be pulled out the memory. Oh yes. Work today. A lot of work.

Trauma in the city shows up in symptoms that are talked about as a ghetto culture. Gun violence between crews is driven by trauma.

The inability to focus at school is trauma too. The drug use and hypersexualization, propelled by trauma. Our kids grow up in war zones. They bear the burden of complex PTSD that one CBS news report called "Hood Disease"; they go numb. They cannot stop seeing their friends die.

Even when a Black or Latino family escapes the barrio and gets one fingernail into the middle class, trauma and its symptoms follow. It changes shape into psychological complexes from impostor syndrome, survivor's guilt, or John Henryism based on the folktale of John Henry, a Black man who drives nails into train tracks. In a race against a steam drill he wins but dies from a heart attack. How many families do I know have elders dead in their fifties and sixties from overwork, hypertension, and alcoholism? Trauma seeps into a new generation and new zip codes, years, even decades after the original pain.

I passed an empty church and thought again of Anderson's essay, the Decent Families versus the Street Families. One reason our kids kill themselves is the institutions that sheltered them are broken. Many Black churches turned to the prosperity gospel that praised wealth and turned Sunday worship into an ATM. Fed up with the hypocrisy, youth fled religion. Many families are fiercely homophobic, yet teens see pop culture embrace gay love. They ran away. For decades now, I have seen a silent migration of queer youth from the Caribbean and the Bible Belt to the Northern cities like New York to escape being gay bashed or killed or forced to live in the closet. The close-knit Black and Latino family that at least compensated conservatism with community has been fractured by social media. During family reunions, people are lost in their little glowing screens as if looking down a well, where one can just make out a reflection at the bottom.

Now "decent" kids are "street" kids too. They run from home like refugees and re-create family in poetry slams or BLM protest marches or youth homeless shelters. None of it is enough. It repeats Émile

Durkheim's 1897 study, *Suicide*. He compared suicide rates of Protestants and Catholics, men and women, single people and those in families. When one floats, untethered by ties to others, be it tradition or love, it is easy to snip the cord of heartbeats that linked one to life. Seventy-six years later, Huey Newton, founder of the Black Panther Party, made that argument in his 1973 memoir, *Revolutionary Suicide*. He defined reactionary suicide as death caused by an inability to fight oppression.

I put the phone away and saw us, here and now, through the many eyes of the many scholars and activists across time. Huey Newton and Émile Durkheim, Coretta Scott King and Ntozake Shange, even the 1989 song "Self Destruction" by the Stop the Violence Movement; all of them saw the same thing. When we are disorganized, fighting each other, spiritually homeless, a people without a direction, a goal, a vision, we wither.

A bus whooshed to the stop. I hurried on. It was nearly empty. I thought of what Lewis wrote in the middle of his essay:

I would cite also a fourth, somewhat speculative example of poverty dissociated from the culture of poverty. [In] Cuba ... I am inclined to believe the culture of poverty does not exist in socialist countries .... In 1947, I undertook a study of a slum in Havana. Recently I had an opportunity to revisit the same slum and some of the same families .... The people were as poor as before but I was impressed to find much less of the feelings of despair and apathy, so symptomatic of the cultures of poverty in the urban slums of the U.S .... The people had found a new sense of power and importance in a doctrine that glorified the lower class as the hope of humanity, and they were armed.

Lewis put a footnote on the role of the slums in social movements. He did not mince words. He came straight for the Left. He wrote,

"The Castro regime—revising Marx and Engels—did not write off the so-called *lumpenproletariat* as an inherently reactionary and anti-revolutionary force but rather found within them a revolutionary potential and utilized it" (24). The potential for change was right here, he said, among the hopeless. If they could see how the ruling class exploited their pain, then their true role in history would shine upon them like a revelation. You are the angels of history.

What now? Lewis wrote that fifty-seven years ago. I googled Fat Joe's interview with Charlamagne tha God on his talk show. Sitting on the couch, he decried the killing of rappers by low-baller thugs as crabs-in-a-barrel shit. At the end, Fat Joe was possessed by the Holy Spirit. The audience grew still. He looked beyond the lights and microphones to a future New York. He steepled his hands, "Let me tell you about Blacks and Latinos, there's no difference between Blacks and Latinos." A woman sitting mid-row snapped her fingers in the air. "You see the same messed up schools, the same hospitals. The biggest power is people power, and if you come together and stop separating the two, you will see the power in numbers would get us exactly what we need in the hood." He chopped the air. "Don't fight your brothers and sisters. We one."

I closed my eyes. The sun shone through the window and warmed me. I heard his last words, "We one." I saw them in my imagination as "We won." In the fight to return to our bodies and to each other. *We won.*

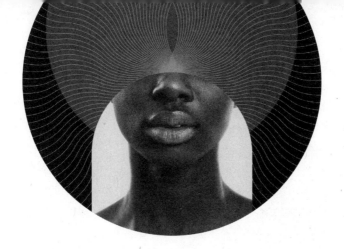

THE HATE THAT HATE PRODUCED

I GOT OFF THE BUS in East Harlem, stood, and asked one question. Where is the Psychedelic Renaissance in the hood? Where is this cutting-edge, futurist community that preaches transformative healing? Where the fuck is everyone? I have been all up and down and not run into one of them.

I see in my email inbox news heralding great results in treating soldiers with PTSD with MDMA. I hear in conferences stories of terminally ill patients who are comforted by psilocybin and hug death like an old friend. I read of depression and addiction cured with psychedelics. Yet here, where kids are shaken by gun violence and Nuyoricans sink into depression and the suicide rate for our teens is going through the roof and nowhere, absolutely nowhere, is a psychedelic organization to be found.

I turn and turn like a spinning bottle. Taino Towers towered above like twin Jenga games built too high and near collapse. In ways I could not always understand, everything here seemed on the edge of collapse. Where was the support? Not far away is Al Sharpton's National Action Network. Downtown is the National Urban League and Hispanic Federation. Midtown hosts the NAACP. Crisscrossing the city, groups advocate for fair housing, criminal justice reform, and immigration. You can knock on their door, ask to talk to someone, check out their program. Maybe join. Yet no psychedelic organizations are doing mass outreach. No leaflets handed out at subway entrances. No pamphlets taped to streetlights. No websites to introduce psychedelics to the hood. No events planned. Nothing to prepare for the upcoming legalization of MDMA as treatment. No protests to push the city to include these new therapies in the tool kit for social workers or in union health care plans.

Turning and turning like a loose hubcap, I see the Taino Towers. Over there is a drunk on the steps of a shuttered store. Over there, yellow police tape fluttered in the wind. Broken glass lay on the sidewalk like teeth punched from a mouth. Where is our second chance?

Maybe we are not ready.

Maybe the thinking in the Psychedelic Renaissance is that there's too much stigma to break through. Sure a few People of Color, mostly middle class, will show up, but overall the masses of people are not going to buy it.

Watching a crowd at the bus stop, faces lit by cellphones. It struck me that drugs are a repeating character in our media. Sitcoms revolve around them like *Breaking Bad* and *Euphoria*, which show drugs as poison or that drugs are freedom.

I heard these stories for years. When I sold weed and LSD in college, it was all about the money. We were businessmen! We played the game but on our own terms. No matter how cool I thought I was, there was always a Person of Color who gave me "The Speech." It was the

"Our People Are Destroyed by Drugs" speech. After they finished, I fanned my face with hundred-dollar bills. Whatever.

I did not want to feel guilt, but I did. Older and more powerful than the Jay-Z school of "I'm not a businessman, I'm a *business*, man" was that drugs are a tool of white supremacy. It was the deep story that framed how we understood drugs in general and psychedelics too. The first time I heard it was, yes, in the finger wagging, "Our People Are Being Destroyed by Crack" speech that Black Nationalist friends used to burn my ears off. The more steeped I became in the history, the further back in time it started.

The first chemical to alter consciousness in the Black Literary Canon was alcohol. In Frederick Douglass's 1845 autobiography, he recalled Christmas holidays when enslavers plied enslaved Blacks with whiskey. He wrote, "It was seen as a disgrace not to get drunk at Christmas." He analyzed how enslavers used drugs as a means to pacify the people:

> From what I know of the effect of these holidays upon the slave, I believe them to be among the most effective means in the hands of the slaveholder in keeping down the spirit of insurrection. Were the slaveholders to abandon this practice, I have not the slightest doubt it would lead to an immediate insurrection among the slaves. These holidays serve as conductors, or safety-valves, to carry off the rebellious spirit of enslaved humanity. (367)

More than one hundred and forty years later, Assata Shakur wrote in her 1988 memoir, *Assata*, a scene with the same warning. She was in the Black Power Movement, visited San Francisco, and got high in the park. It was just weed but strong weed. She was zonked and did not see cops sweeping the park, arresting Hippies and activists. Assata wrote:

> I was feeling guilty and stupid, silly and politically backward. I was embarrassed to be bumbling down the street in the middle of the day

and not in full control of my faculties, too high to deal with reality much less change it. . . . It was obvious my stuff was raggedy and that I needed to get my act together. If I wanted to call myself a revolutionary I was going to have to earn the title. I had heard somebody say that revolutionaries get high on the revolution and that it was the best high in the world. "I'm gonna check out that high," I said aloud. (202)

The theme tying Frederick Douglass and Assata to preachers and Black Nationalists is that drugs are a tool of white supremacy. They blur our senses. They dull our brains. Drugs are chemical chains, clamped on neurons so we cannot imagine freedom much less act free. They trap us on the plantation. Not just the real historical one in the antebellum era but the plantation that persists throughout time that changes into new forms like twentieth-century sharecropping, prisons, and ghettos.

Standing in Spanish Harlem, knowing the headlines of fentanyl busts in a Bronx childcare center and killer drug crews, it was clear some of us became chemical overseers. Using the plantation as a metaphor meant asking, What new chains do we wear? Who owns us? Who works for the owners? In that lens, white overseers from the antebellum era were replaced by Black and Latino men who sold drugs to us in order to enrich themselves. What small freedom they achieved was financed by our destruction.

The betrayal caused rage at drug dealers as combustible as nitroglycerin. I remember the antidrug speech in films like 1991's *New Jack City* and *Ricochet*, when the Black leading man, usually Denzel Washington, confronted dealers with "What the fuck is wrong with y'all? Selling dope to each other. 'Cause that's all you're doing. 'Cause you damn sure ain't selling no drug over in Beverly Hills." You saw it in the early '90s TV show *Roc* starring burly actor Charles S. Dutton who squared off with a local drug kingpin as the neighborhood rallied behind him. The Hollywood slick scenes of a final confrontation between a Decent Man and a Street Man were fantasy. Real life is not tidy. What it did represent was a pent-up desire to kill the new overseers, who used chemicals instead of whips. Who were Black and Latino, not white. The enemy had changed face and color but was an enemy, nevertheless.

The Plantation Metaphor is so powerful, so energized with emotion that even a scientist will hit a brick wall. I pulled up on my phone the heated interview Dr. Carl Hart had on Power 105.1's morning show, *The Breakfast Club*, hosted by DJ Envy, Charlamagne tha God, and until recently, Angela Yee. Hart is a scientist. The brother ran tests on drug addiction for decades, wrote numerous books, and repeatedly hit one point. Most drug users do not fit the Drug War stereotype where if you take one hit from the "glass dick," you transform into a homeless, scabies-having, trick-turning crackhead.

Hart discovered most drug users are regular shmegular, working peeps who do blow sometimes, weed sometimes, maybe do a bounce of heroin or special k and then work or pick up kids from daycare. Nearly 70 percent of users are normal everyday folks, part of the endless flow of faces on the morning commute. In his research, backed up by others, actual drug addiction is less about the chemical in this or that narcotic than of deeper problems like trauma and social inequality.

So, that did not go over well. Within minutes of the show, Charlamagne began to get in his ass. In. His. Ass.

"I'm watching your body language, and I see you shaking." He verbally poked Hart. "I'm asking myself, Is he going through withdrawal?"

Hart's face scrunched up. "C'mon man."

The camera zoomed in. Hart threw a dismissive hand as if tossing a dirty napkin. DJ Envy and Charlamagne needled him with Drug War propaganda. Hart kept putting on the table his vision. Let us have testing centers so no one gets a hot needle or bad batch. Let us regulate drugs to end their stigma. I knew Hart's story from other interviews and documentaries. The man had been trappin' in Miami. He dealt drugs. He got out the game. He studied and trained and ran tests. At first he was pro Drug War until he looked at the data provided by his own experiments. The results inexorably moved him to reconsider a whole generation of government propaganda. Now, he invokes the Black prophetic tradition, yes, the MLK, Frederick Douglass, Ella Baker, Coretta Scott King tradition of calling for the embrace of the outcast, except now, the outcast is the drug user.

I shut the phone off and sighed. How the hell do psychedelics break through that stigma? How does LSD or MDMA or mushrooms become a cure for us?

An immense healing is at our fingertips, but it is not being introduced to us. The risk is that even if it were, we still might condemn it as another Tuskegee experiment. Our pain over pain is so deep, we may trust it more than healing.

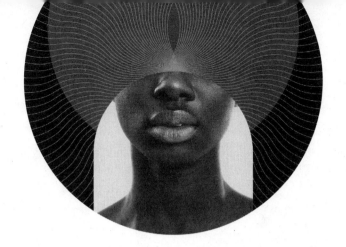

THE BEAUTYFUL ONES ARE NOT YET BORN

MAYBE THERE IS NO HOPE.

I turned and turned like a compass needle in empty space. Where does one go? On the side of a building, a mural caught my eye. An artist painted a mother holding her baby, inside the Freedom Tower. The skyscraper's triangle glass and steel encased her like a suit of armor. Did it mean the Freedom Tower was a symbol of the city's rebirth after 9/11? Did it mean we need to protect our children, our future, from terrorism?

Old grief filled my throat. One thing I know is when pain breaks you, the pieces can be put back, but it reshapes you. It was not just me. All over New York, I saw tiny remembrances of 9/11; framed photos of the Twin Towers on delis and pizza places, a Never Forget decal on a firetruck, a Twin Tower logo on a hat or T-shirt. There were a lot less now than before; I mean, it had been twenty years.

History is a race between trauma and healing. For us, the Freedom Tower was a symbol of our resurrection. We were not going to live in fear. We could heal and move on, not just from 9/11 but Hurricane Sandy, Covid, and Trump. Jolted by the mural, I began to walk. Some instinct told me to go to the Freedom Tower. It was our compass needle. It would help me figure out this question of hope.

I made my way down Lexington Avenue. If psychedelic therapy is going to be part of our lives, our city, our culture again, who will it be for? How will it be introduced so that it goes beyond costly treatments here or pricey New Age getaways in Mexico or Costa Rica? How does it build enough of a base to overcome the inevitable Conservative reaction? How can it lead to revolution?

The Medical Model's Trojan horse strategy made sense. Start as life-saving treatment for those who saved our lives. New Yorkers know city workers deserve it. After 9/11, we saw photos of dust-coated cops and firefighters at Ground Zero. During Covid, the media showed nurses and doctors, faces bruised from wearing masks for days as they treated the sick. When frontline workers came home, we hit pots and pans together, hailing them as heroes.

Yet I knew from conversations over the years that our heroes were in pain. On the corner, a garbage truck puttered as men hauled black bags into the back. I remembered a year ago seeing a sanitation worker with a heavy sadness. I asked, "You good?" He blurted out that his friend got nailed by a piece of metal thrown in the trash. It was bent by the truck's hydraulic press and snapped, sailed through the air and hit the man's chest like a spear, exploding his heart. He shook his head. He said he knew guys that accidentally breathed chemicals thrown in the trash and lost their lungs. "People don't know." He stared at me. "They don't know."

I imagine him on the garbage truck in front of me now. The LSD is a paintbrush, and in a few blinks an imaginary scene takes shape. I daydream him in the front seat, checking his cell to confirm an appointment. He reads a dog-eared pamphlet. On it is the acronym TRIP—Therapeutic Restoration Informed by Psychedelics. The glossy cover shows an MTA employee in a recliner and wearing an eye mask. He thumbs the page, and inside, Governor Kathy Hochul introduces the new treatment available through union health insurance.

At the end of his shift, he showers and rides the bus to a Midtown clinic. He pushes the glass doors, signs in, and is taken to a circle of city workers on chairs. A subway emergency team worker talks about scooping up the bits and pieces of a jumper crushed by a train. A cop stammers as she tells of picking up from the floor teeth from a woman battered by her husband. An EMT says he had nightmares of being trapped in the ambulance, unable to leave as people bled on the sidewalk.

One by one, a nurse leads them to a private room to lie on a mat and gives them a dose of MDMA. Euphoria fills the sanitation worker like helium. Floating above himself, he sees his friend hit by the steel beam. He yanks it free and tells his buddy to take the day off. They agree it is time to demand safer trucks. The MDMA fades. When he takes off the eye mask, dried tears are on his face, but he feels lighter, freer.

He tells his coworkers who tease him at first but then hug him, say congrats, and ruffle his hair. They go home and tell friends and family. One by one, city workers who get psychedelic therapy share their stories, which trickle into families, friends, and flow into neighborhoods.

Word spreads. Whatever this psychedelic thing is, it works. I imagine that man I met on this garbage truck smiling as he pushes the hydraulic press. I want that for him. He deserves it. They all deserve it. In this LSD fantasy, I imagine that at the end of the shift, he hops off the truck and starts to walk to the Freedom Tower. MTA workers emerge from subway stations and smile in new peacefulness. Cops, firefighters, and teachers join a march of civil servants healed by psychedelic therapy. They bring the authority of city workers who carry eight million people on their shoulders.

The LSD peeled reality apart. It pulled from the living breathing people in front of me, one possible future like a sheet of cellophane. The other reality crinkled in bright vivid colors. I saw two worlds. I knew one was real. I knew the other was only a dream. But it was so close I could touch it.

What if psychedelic therapy were available to social workers? I imagine clients who stand at the doors of a treatment center nervously holding the TRIP pamphlet. The case manager takes their hand and says it is going to be okay. They guide the client to a low-lit room with ocean sounds. Fidgety, one woman, thin and scarred, sits on a warm mat. She talks about binge drinking and fistfighting her boyfriend. The more the story unspools, the further back in time it goes until she talks with her father, who left the family.

The social worker gives her psilocybin. The client wears an eye mask and from her unconscious rises sharp grief. Behind closed eyes, a dim patch of color moves toward her and takes the shape of her father. He seems to walk on bioluminescent water, every footfall stirring glowing trails. The closer he gets, years peel off his face. He becomes a teen, a child, then a baby. She cradles him. A mirror faces her. In it she sees that her reflection is her grandfather. The old man had been jailed and never saw his son, her father, the baby in her arms. He never saw her either. The reflections fall on each other like dominoes on a table. Pushed by the pain of abandonment.

The psilocybin wears off. The client tears off the eye mask and sees the long, winding path that trauma takes in her family's life. She palms her chest and feels her heart kick and says over and over, "I understand."

Imagine her leaving the treatment center and joining the MTA workers, cops, sanitation crews, paramedics, and firefighters. Client after client opens the center doors and stops to look in wonder at their hands. They study fingers and wrists and palms in wonder. They touch their faces, then each other's faces as if they were beautiful sculptures by Rodin.

The growing throng studies their arms and faces. They gather in the street, on stoops and intersections. They hold each other like reunited lovers. They have returned to their bodies. Euphoria gives way to sadness. Why were they separated from themselves for so long? Who dulled them to the painful beauty all around them? The air—my god—was it always electric? Was breathing always filled with so much flavor?

Gathering in parks, feeling grass tickle fingertips, workers rejoice in the world. Every touch feels like a miracle. Songs burst from mouths like roses. No one knows who began it but pressing palms with another person becomes a greeting. A new image rises from the warm, tactile communion. The Body, they keep talking about the Body as what everyone has in common and is older than ideology or theology. Across the city, Collective Transference charges the air like static before a storm. Hair rises on the back of people's necks. Whole groups take LSD and press palms. They stare at and touch their limbs as if they were just born.

While I was walking down Lexington Avenue, the LSD made it easy to see what the future can be. Each wave of psychedelic therapy must smash an invisible wall separating the deserving from the undeserving. Of course, workers deserve it. We owe them our world. So do the sick. They did not cause their illness. What about ex-felons? What of the chronic poor? Do they deserve a second chance?

Imagine an ex-felon going to a freshly painted treatment center with a crumpled TRIP pamphlet in his back pocket. His brother, who drives a bus for the city, told him psychedelic therapy worked and he should sign up. It comes with time off parole, less check-ins. He is like fuck it, why not. He saunters into the treatment center, slaps the pamphlet on the desk, boom-shouts he is here for the Hippie shit. The staff look at each other, smile, and usher him to his therapist. The doctor is a salt-and-pepper-haired Black man with bright red glasses and a boxer's broken nose. He sizes up the client and asks him to walk and talk.

The two men joke about jail; they had both done time. They shake heads at the transition to civilian life. Finally the therapist asks if he saw his son. The man snaps no. They meet over weeks, undressing old wounds, and the therapist even has the client sit on different chairs and talk from the perspective of his father, his son, his baby mama, and finally himself as a child. After two months, the therapist takes him to a candlelit room and the client lies on a thick mat, swallows the LSD, and holds a photo of himself kissing his newborn son, nine years ago. The LSD strips husk from mind. The tough-guy act and loudness slide off. The more he looks at the photo, the more it moves like film. In it, his face changes into his son's face. The newborn's face changes into his middle-aged face. They have reversed roles, and his son now cradles his father, says the same thing he said nine years ago in the hospital, "I waited for you my whole life."

The LSD ebbs like low tide. The ex-felon presses the photo to his chest, snot bubbles from his nose while apologizing. Days later, he goes to the basketball court where his son plays and waits. His palms are sweaty. He knows the kid will diss him. They had not seen each other in years. He is a failure. What child will want him? The boy dribbles with his friends, sees his father, and turns absentmindedly to a teammate, spins back, and yells. He runs and his father catches him. They fall to the ground and weep and sway back and forth.

Imagine him walking out of the housing projects, holding his son's hand and joining the massive march of MTA and sanitation workers, cops and firefighters, social workers and their clients, paramedics and their patients. Hundreds of thousands fill the avenue like a river. Heads rise and fall like waves. Voices swell and sizzle like seafoam. A vision glows in their faces as if the sun shines on every one of them.

At each housing project the march passes, men and women pour from the buildings. They shake the streets. The Section 8 houses are brightened by art. Murals make walls into utopian visions. Graffiti artists paint snapped slave chains that morph into a DNA double-helix that becomes ladders climbed by children into a clean futuristic New York. Flowers are painted on trash cans. Poetry is written in mul-ticolored chalk on the sidewalk. In playgrounds, activists announce the new Exodus. Standing on top of the jungle gym, they shout through a megaphone that "trauma cuts us from our bodies, our his-tory and city." They raised the volume: "The Black Freedom Struggle has always been returning to our truth." Holding the Bible and the Circle Seven Koran and the real Koran, they dramatically throw them into the trash. "We do not need lies. No more gods. No more masters. Our bodies are the holy text. Our bodies are the promised land."

Imagine in the most blood-soaked neighborhoods psychedelic strike teams of violence interrupters take rival gangs to the African Burial Ground. They sit them face-to-face, give them MDMA. Thera-pists ask them to tell their enemies about the person they killed. Who were they? Why did you love them? Why do you miss them? Stories rebound through the night. Stripped raw by the MDMA, they real-ize the man they killed was just like them. "I'm sorry," one says, then another. "I'm sorry." They wipe tears with gang bandannas. They look at the monument, sigh, and feel the ancestors buried inside them. They reach for each other, and say, "Never again. By any means necessary."

A joyous New York rises from the dead husk of the old New York. Hundreds of thousands flood the streets. In their eyes is a burning question: How did we get so low? How did we get used to our own depravity? Why did everyone forget we are human? Why did we? In a seesaw effect, crime plummets to near zero as protests erupt. Vowing not to go back, mi gente stage die-ins at banks, occupy city hall; crowds block traffic and chant. They demand better housing, better schools, and jobs.

The mayor orders the police to crack down. Only a third show up in riot gear. The rest are too moved by the beauty to crush it. Many have seen the healing up close and cannot kill it. A threadbare line of cops stands in the avenue like a cheap necklace. They try to stop the river of New Yorkers. Face-to-face with colleagues they have known their whole lives. Hands tremble on batons. Friends in sanitation or doctors or social workers gently push aside the riot shields. They fall on the ground like large fingernail clippings.

The governor on TV calls for law and order. The TRIP program is canceled, but it is too late. Activists organize a Psychedelic Underground Railroad where secret meetings take place in safe spaces to continue radical therapy. New language grows from the navel like an umbilical cord to instinctual truths. Abandoned offices are repurposed for LSD consciousness raising. Odd combos show up, a middle-aged doorman, a subway driver, a sex worker, and migrants. They lie on mats, and on psychedelics, dig through a kaleidoscope unconscious. Afterward, they sit up and see the strangers they came in with are now bathed in a new light. Each pair of eyes, a mirror to their own depths. They share different languages, how their lives were pulped in the gears of modern life. Wealth wrung from them to create power for the powerful.

I am so lost in imagining psychedelic New York that I do not realize how far I walked. I am across the street from Madison Square Garden. It is lit up and buzzed with people going in for an event. Standing outside a deli, nurses on lunch gossip and smoke cigarettes. A Chinese man fixes the mannequin in a store window. Whoever I see is split in two, the flesh-and-blood person, yes, but also, as if peeling off plastic wrapping, who they could be shimmers in the air. In this dreamed-up city, the lines of people that pour into the stadium carry Fat Joe for Mayor signs. Speakers boom the speech he gives inside. I hear his nasal Bronx voice yelling in rap cadence that it is time for workers to go "all the way up." Thunderous foot stomping and yelling and roars make the sidewalk vibrate.

Why did I think this movement could be different? Why does a worker-led Psychedelic Revolution succeed where the '68 generation failed? The secret is it does not need a Moral Shock to get us "woke." When done right. When done with the proper Set, Setting, and Container, the masses taste Heaven. The people experience the transcendent interconnectedness with each other and themselves and their bodies. With that euphoria at hand, the joy and love for another world fuel the movement.

The Psychedelic Renaissance becomes the Psychedelic Revolution when it serves the multiracial working class. It really is that simple. When workers win, everyone wins. I turn the corner with a tornado of butterflies in my head. Down the avenue is the Freedom Tower. I put in earbuds and play Roberta Flack's "The First Time Ever I Saw Your Face" and people-watch. The New York I conjured on my LSD trip seems loony. Most would say it does not exist, but I saw it. I lived it. After 9/11, we searched photos of the dead with candles and held hands at bars. We listened to each other's loss. I lived with it in quarantine when Covid put the city into a forced coma and we wore masks to save lives. I marched with it during Occupy Wall Street and Black Lives Matter. Every day when buildings caught fire or we got sick or kids shot kids, I saw our best—civil servants risking their lives for strangers even when it was hopeless. Even when it cost their own lives.

We live in two New Yorks. One rough and greedy. One luminous with love and courage. You have to live here a while to see both cities wrapped inside each other. When a crisis hits, the people's soul burns the thin screen that separates them. Sometimes we look away. We have been warned for decades not to stare at bright lights. Think of Times Square. You get blinded. You get hustled. Yet our love for each other rises like towers of light. If we saw without blinking. If we touched it. We would know how powerful and handsome we are. We could change ourselves. We could change the world.

EPILOGUE

The party rages. Outside the Freedom Tower it is like the scene from *The Wiz*. Dancers leap and twist. Police cars blare deep house music. Buses rock as passengers sway side to side. Passersby toss beers to them. A huge bonfire paints the skyscrapers red and gold. Thousands encircle it, drumming, and chanting. Climbing on top of a turned-over jeep, I can see the streets filled with jumping, thrashing, raucous New York.

I walk to the Freedom Tower. Inside the hall is empty. I see the celebration from the other side of closed doors. The elevator light is on. I enter and feel the g-force as it shoots up, up, up to the observatory deck. It stops. Doors open.

Wind and clouds whip my clothes. Buffeted, I grip the rail. No windows? No one here? The observatory deck is abandoned. The circular hall wraps the Freedom Tower, and I see New York. The sky flows in and rocks me like a kite. Clouds fill the hall; I stumble in the vaporous fog. Damp paper smacks my face. I pull it off and see that it is a page from this book. Tearing more down, each one is another page. The walls are made of reams of pages. I want to leave but the elevator is gone.

"Thank you," a voice calls.

I see my son. He is full grown. The same green-brown eyes. The same mischievous ferret smile. He takes my elbow, and in the window's reflection I'm old and frail.

"Thank you for writing this book."

"Where are we?" I clutch him.

"The end." He kisses my forehead. "Now it is my story. You wrote this to give me a chance. The book is flawed." He pats me like a child. "Melodramatic. Pretentious. But you gave us a vision. Now we can imagine a way to survive." He escorts me to the ledge. "Listen."

I crane my neck. Wind carries voices from across the planet. No bombs. No guns. No parents crying over dead children. No war. No hunger. I hear peace. The sun flashes, and I blink tears.

"How?"

"That's for my generation to worry about." He hugs me. "I love you." He lifts my wrinkled body up like a trophy. Wind scatters feet and hands, arms, and legs. In the clouds, I see Mom and Dad, my grandparents, and ancestors. I am loved. The last gust blasts me into pieces, and I spin into the sky. Up. Up. Up.

the brightness

the brightness!

REFERENCES

Alexander, Michelle. *The New Jim Crow*. New York: The New Press, 2012.

Alpert, Richard. "The LSD Crisis." YouTube video. April 16, 2011. www
.youtube.com/watch?v=7P3TrGCMHNU&t=111s.

Anderson, Elijah. "The Code of the Streets." *The Atlantic*, May 1994, 86.

Aptheker, Herbert. *American Negro Slave Revolts*. New York: Columbia
Press, 1943.

Baldwin, James. "No Name in the Street," in *The Price of the Ticket*, 547.
New York: St. Martin's Press, 1985.

Baraka, Amiri. *The LeRoi Jones/Amiri Baraka Reader*. New York: Thun-
dermouth Press, 1991.

Blassingame, John. *The Slave Community: Plantation Life in the Antebellum South*. New York: Oxford University Press, 1979.

Borowski, Tadeusz. *This Way to the Gas, Ladies and Gentlemen*. 1946.
New York: Penguin, 1992.

Caldwell, W. V. *LSD Psychotherapy: An Exploration of Psychedelic and
Psycholytic Therapy*. New York: Grove Press, 1968.

Cesaire, Aime. *A Discourse on Colonialism*. New York: Monthly Review
Press, 1950.

Cleaver, Kathleen. "Kathleen Cleaver and Natural Hair." YouTube
video. August 2, 2014. www.youtube.com/watch?v=LWbIHcm6xSc.

Collins, Patricia Hill. *Black Feminist Thought*. New York: Routledge, 2009.

Columbus, Christopher. *The Four Voyages of Christopher Columbus*.
Translated and Edited by J. M. Cohen. New York: Penguin, 1969.

Cosby, Bill. "Pound Cake Speech." NAACP Legal Defense Fund Awards Ceremony, Washington DC, May 17, 2004. YouTube video. www.youtube.com/watch?v=CG5r5ByCbMI.

Cross, William E. "The Negro-to-Black Conversion Experience." *Black World*, July 1971, 82–83.

Dangerfield, George. *The Strange Death of Liberal England*. New York: Smith and Hass, 1935.

Dass, Ram. *Be Here Now*. San Cristobal, NM: The Lama Foundation, 1971.

De Beauvoir, Simone. "The Second Sex." In *The Norton Anthology of Theory and Criticism*. Edited by Vincent B. Leitch, 1403. New York: W. W. Norton, 2001.

Didion, Joan. *Slouching Towards Bethlehem*. New York: Farrar, Straus and Giroux, 1961.

Dillon, Michele. *Introduction to Sociological Theory*. Sussex, UK: Wiley-Blackwell, 2010.

Doblin, Rick. "Net Zero Trauma." YouTube video. April 21, 2021. www.youtube/watch?v=H8ULBNiev7s.

Doblin, Rick. "Regulation of the Medical Use of Psychedelics and Marijuana." PhD diss., Harvard University, 2000.

Douglass, Frederick. "Narrative of the Life of Frederick Douglass." In *The Norton Anthology of African American Literature*. Edited by Henry Louis Gates Jr. and Nellie Y. McKay, 395. New York: W. W. Norton, 2004.

Du Bois, W. E. B. *Black Reconstruction*. New York: The Free Press, 1962.

Du Bois, W. E. B. "The Souls of Black Folk." In *The Norton Anthology of African American Literature*. Edited by Henry Louis Gates Jr. and Nellie Y. McKay, 694. New York: W. W. Norton, 2004.

Dunbar, Paul Laurence. "We Wear the Mask." In *The Norton Anthology of African American Literature*. Edited by Henry Louis Gates Jr. and Nellie Y. McKay. New York: W. W. Norton, 2004.

Durkheim, Émile. *Suicide*. New York: Routledge, 2005.

Emery, Lynne Fauley. *Black Dance: From 1619 to Today.* Princeton, NJ: Princeton Book Co., 1989.

Fanon, Frantz. *The Wretched of the Earth.* New York: Grove Press, 1961.

Frazier, E. Franklin. "The Pathology of Race Prejudice." *Forum Magazine* LXXVII, no. 6 (1927): 856–62.

Freud, Sigmund. "Group Psychology and the Analysis of the Ego." In *Great Books of the Western World,* Vol. 54, Edited by Mortimer J. Adler, 666. Chicago: Encyclopedia Britannica, 1952.

Ginsberg, Allen. *Howl and Other Poems.* New York: City Lights, 1956.

Hart, Carl, and Charles Ksir. *Drugs, Society and Human Behavior,* 16th ed. New York: McGraw-Hill, 2015.

Harvey, David. "Capital Volume One: Capital in Motion." YouTube video. September 30, 2016. www.youtube.com/watch?v=4MceeO4Ulrs.

Hegel, Georg Wilhelm Friedrich. *Phenomenology of Spirit.* Translated by A. V. Miller. New York: Oxford University Press, 1977.

Hinckle, Warren. "The Social History of Hippies," in *Ransoming Pagan Babies: The Selected Writings of Warren Hinckle.* Berkeley, CA: Heyday Publishing, 2018.

Hitchens, Christopher. "Is There a Liberal Crack-Up?" *Firing Line* by William Buckley, 1984. YouTube video. www.youtube.com /@HooverLibraryArchives.

Hoffman, Alfred. *LSD: My Problem Child.* New York: McGraw Hill, 1979.

Hortogsohn, Ido. *American Trip: Set and Setting and the Psychedelic Experience in the Twentieth Century.* Cambridge, MA: MIT Press, 2020.

Hurston, Zora Neale. "Characteristics of Negro Expressions." In *The Norton Anthology of African American Literature.* Edited by Henry Louis Gates Jr. and Nellie Y. McKay, 1049. New York: W. W. Norton, 2004.

Hurston, Zora Neale. "How It Feels to Be Colored Me," in *The Norton Anthology of African American Literature.* Edited by Henry Louis Gates Jr. and Nellie Y. McKay, 1032. New York: W. W. Norton, 2004.

Huxley, Aldous. *Brave New World*. 1932. Reprinted New York: Harper Perennial, 2006.

Huxley, Aldous. *The Doors of Perception*. 1954. Reprinted New York: Harper Perennial, 2009.

James, C. L. R. *The Black Jacobins: Toussaint L'Ouverture and the San Domingo Revolution*. New York: Random House, 1963.

Jarecki, Eugene, dir. *The House I Live In*. 2013. New York: Charlotte Street Films.

Jarnow, Jesse. *Heads*. Boston: De Capo Press, 2009.

Jasper, James. *The Art of Moral Protest*. Chicago: University of Chicago Press, 1999.

Joe, Fat. "Death of a Democracy," Episode 6, *Hell of a Week with Charlamagne Da God*. Video. Paramount, September 15, 2022. www.paramountplus.com/shows/video/poeAozocssWs2uD_qoY _rgmBZ2YIxdHK.

King, Martin Luther, Jr. "Letter from a Birmingham Jail." In *The Norton Anthology of African American Literature*. Edited by Henry Louis Gates Jr. and Nellie Y. McKay, 1895. New York: W. W. Norton, 2004.

Laplanche, Jean, and Jean-Bertrand Pontalis. *The Language of Psycho-Analysis*. New York: W. W. Norton, 1973.

Las Casas, Bartolomé. *A Short Account of the Destruction of the Indies*. Translated by Nigel Griffin. New York: Penguin Classics, 1999.

Lewis, Oscar. "The Culture of Poverty." *Scientific American* 15, no. 4 (1966): 19.

Lukács, György. "Realism in the Balance." In *The Norton Anthology of Theory and Criticism*. Edited by Vincent B. Leitch, 1033–37. New York: W. W. Norton, 2001.

Marcuse, Herbert. *One-Dimensional Man*. Boston: Beacon Press, 1991.

Marx, Karl. "Economic Manuscripts of 1844." In *The Marx-Engels Reader*. Edited by Robert C. Tucker, 72. New York: W. W. Norton, 1978.

Marx, Karl. "Manifesto of the Communist Party." In *The Marx-Engels Reader*. Edited by Robert C. Tucker, 473–74. New York: W. W. Norton, 1978.

McKenna, Terrance. *Food of the Gods*. New York: Bantam, 1993.

Mills, C. Wright. *The Power Elite*. Oxford, UK: Oxford University Press, 1975.

Morrison, Toni. *Beloved*. New York: Vintage Books, 1987.

Mosley, Tonya. "Letting Go." *Truth Be Told*. Podcast. April 20, 2023. https://pod.link/1462216572/episode/2a88c9a46c775e4d9c6f191b48b72796.

National Geographic. *The Visual History of the World*. Washington, DC: National Geographic Society, 2005.

Newton, Huey. *Revolutionary Suicide*. New York: Penguin, 2009.

Obama, Barack. *Audacity of Hope*. New York: Broadway Books, 2007.

Pollan, Michael. *How to Change Your Mind*. New York: Penguin, 2018.

Pryor, Richard. *Pryor Convictions*. New York: Amistad Books, 1995.

Rilke, Rainer Maria. *The Notebooks of Malte Laurids Brigge*. Translated by Michael Hulse. London: Penguin, 2009.

Rimbaud, Arthur. "Letter." In *The Norton Anthology of Theory and Criticism*. Edited by Vincent B. Leitch, 1871. New York: W. W. Norton, 2001.

Rock, Chris. "Chris Rock, Truth, Therapy and Punchline." *CBS Sunday Morning by Gayle Jones*. January 3, 2021. www.cbs.com/shows/video/tHL_7PoQlylP_UraDoKdFCrBgeuRdaB8.

Roy, Sriparna, and Mariam E Sunny. "US FDA Declines to Approve First MDMA-based PTSD Treatment." www.reuters.com, August 10, 2024. Accessed August 14, 2024. https://www.reuters.com/business/healthcare-pharmaceuticals/us-fda-declines-approve-first-mdma-based-ptsd-treatment-2024-08-09/.US

Shakur, Assata. *Assata: An Autobiography*. New York: Lawrence Hill Books, 1988.

Shange, Ntozake. *For Colored Girls Who Have Considered Suicide When the Rainbow Is Enuf*. New York: Scribner, 2010.

Siculus, Diodorus. "The First Slave War on the Island of Sicily." In *Spartacus and the Slave Wars: A Brief History with Documents.* Translated and edited by Brent D. Shaw, 80. Boston: St. Martin's Press, 2001.

Siegel, Larry J. *Criminology.* Belmont, CA: Thomson Wadsworth, 2009.

Smith, Will. "Will Smith's Red Table Talk Take-Over." *Red Table Talk. By Will Smith and Dr. Ramani Durvasula.* Video. November 20, 2020. www.facebook.com/redtabletalk/videos/3823074501060289.

Spitzer, Robert L., ed. *Diagnostic and Statistical Manual of Mental Disorders,* 3rd ed. Washington, DC: American Psychiatric Association, 1985.

Stevens, Jay. *Storming Heaven.* New York: Grove Press, 1998.

Thomas, Piri. *Down These Mean Streets.* 1967. Reprinted New York: Vintage, 1997.

Thompson, Hunter S. *Fear and Loathing in Las Vegas.* 1972. Reprinted New York: Vintage, 1998.

Thompson, Hunter S. *Hell's Angels.* 1967. Reprinted New York: Random House, 1991.

Touré. *Who's Afraid of Post-Blackness.* New York: Atria Books, 1991.

Wollstonecraft, Mary. "A Vindication of the Rights of Women." In *The Norton Anthology of Theory and Criticism.* Edited by Vincent B. Leitch, 1792. New York: W. W. Norton, 2001.

X, Malcolm. *The Autobiography of Malcolm X.* New York: Random House, 1964.

INDEX

I

ibogaine, xviii, 167–168
Imara, Kufikiri, xvii
Immersion/Immersion-Emersion
  stage, Negro-to-Black Conversion
  Experience, 21, 29, 85
impostor syndrome, 200
infanticide, Hippies, 128
informal integration, 7
insurance coverage, 67
integration, 6–7, 10
Integration, Structural Functionalism,
  115
intergenerational trauma, xiv, xviii
Internalization stage, Negro-to-Black
  Conversion Experience, 21, 29
internalized racism, 22, 33, 77
"Internalized Racism's Association with
  African American Male Youth's
  Propensity for Violence" (Bryant), 199
Introduction to Sociological Theory
  (Dillon), 114
Iraq War, 5

J

J. P. Morgan, 142
Jama-Everett, Ayize, xvii
Jamaican Rasta, 36
Jarnow, Jesse, 112
Jasper, James
  The Art of Moral Protest, 83
  The Black Jacobins, 84
  Moral Shock, 85
Jay-Z, 138, 205
The Jeffersons, 33, 182
Jesus Christ Superstar, xix
John Henryism, 200
John Hopkins University, 142
John, Elton, 192
Jones, Precious, 192
jook joints, 74
joy, 84, 86
Juneteenth, 84

K

Kenney, Jim, 40
Kenya, 18–21, 23–24, 27
Kesey, Ken, 128
ketamine, PTSD, 47, 50
Keys, Alicia, 138
King, Coretta Scott, 201
King, Gayle, 9
King, Martin Luther Jr., 23
  assassination, 83, 86
Klein, Melanie, 45
Knocked Up, 130
Koran, 215
Korean War, 117
Kubrick, Stanley, 19
Kubrin, Charis E., 199
kykeon, xviii

L

Lacan, Jacques, 45
Lamar, Kendrick, 37
Lang, Fritz, 194
The Language of Psycho-Analysis
  (Laplanche and Pontalis), xxi, 67, 71,
  123, 124
Laplanche, Jean, xxi, 67, 71, 123
Latifah, Queen, xvii
Latinos, 184, 187, 192, 197, 200, 202, 207
Leary, Timothy, 117–119, 129
legality, xviii, 65–66, 100, 135
  criminalization of LSD, 120–121
  criminalization of psychedelics,
    128–129
  psychedelic therapy, 76
legalization, 56–57, 111
The LeRoi Jones / Amiri Baraka Reader, 84
"Letter from Birmingham Jail" (King
  Jr.), 23
Lewis, Oscar, 195–196, 201–202
liberalism, 133
Life magazine, 167
Little, Malcolm, 70, 72. *See also* Malcolm X
Live on the Sunset Strip (Pryor), 18, 20

ABOUT THE AUTHOR

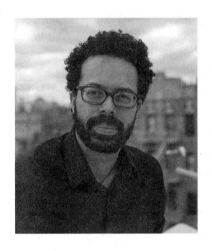

Dr. Nicholas Powers, PhD, is a novelist, poet, and journalist living in New York. He is a tenured associate professor of literature at SUNY Old Westbury, where his courses include topics ranging from African American literature, creative nonfiction, and Black women writers to literature of class consciousness, autobiography, and literature across cultures.

Never one to shy away from a hot take, Dr. Powers's political writing has appeared in *Truth-Out, The Indypendent, The Catalyst, Raw Story, Business Insider, Lucid News, The Village Voice,* and *Vibe.* He has presented talks and reported from the Psychedelic Renaissance since 2017, starting with his talk at the 2017 Horizons Conference. Since then, he has written for numerous psychedelic publications including *Lucid News* and *Double Blind* and has given talks at Naropa University and Chacruna Institute for Psychedelic Research.

In addition to being involved in the Psychedelic Renaissance, Dr. Powers has published three books with Upset Press: *Thirst,* a political vampire novel; *The Ground Below Zero,* a mix of reportage from disaster zones, protests, and Burning Man; and published in 2013, *Theater of War, a* collection of poetry.

Dr. Powers attended *Wild Seeds Writers Retreat* and the *Cave Canem* Black poetry workshops regularly. In 2024, he will lead the memoir workshop at *Wild Seeds Writers Retreat*. He also co-hosted, with poet Christine Timm, the NYC College Slam at the Nuyorican Poets Café from 2014 to 2022.

ABOUT NORTH ATLANTIC BOOKS

North Atlantic Books (NAB) is an independent, nonprofit publisher committed to a bold exploration of the relationships between mind, body, spirit, and nature. Founded in 1974, NAB aims to nurture a holistic view of the arts, sciences, humanities, and healing. To make a donation or to learn more about our books, authors, events, and newsletter, please visit www.north atlanticbooks.com.